Haifa MTIR

Mediastinitis following cardiac surgery

Haifa MT IR

Mediastinitis following cardiac surgery

Predictors of mortality

ScienciaScripts

Imprint

Any brand names and product names mentioned in this book are subject to trademark, brand or patent protection and are trademarks or registered trademarks of their respective holders. The use of brand names, product names, common names, trade names, product descriptions etc. even without a particular marking in this work is in no way to be construed to mean that such names may be regarded as unrestricted in respect of trademark and brand protection legislation and could thus be used by anyone.

Cover image: www.ingimage.com

This book is a translation from the original published under ISBN 978-620-6-72564-0.

Publisher:
Sciencia Scripts
is a trademark of
Dodo Books Indian Ocean Ltd. and OmniScriptum S.R.L publishing group

120 High Road, East Finchley, London, N2 9ED, United Kingdom
Str. Armeneasca 28/1, office 1, Chisinau MD-2012, Republic of Moldova, Europe
Printed at: see last page
ISBN: 978-3-330-33611-7

Contents

1 INTRODUCTION

The approach to the anterior mediastinum via a vertical median sternotomy and its osteosynthesis with steel wires at the end of the operation was first described by Milton in 1897. It was not until 1956 that M.Julian presented it as the approach of choice in cardiac surgery(I).

The sternum is the cornerstone of thoracic dynamics. Subject to constant post-operative stress (movement, breathing, coughing), the sternotomy is an area of thoracic instability, and therefore fragility, with a high risk of scarring complications(2).

Post-cardiac surgery mediastinitis is a deep infection of the surgical site, and includes involvement of tissues above the subcutaneous level, i.e. sternal osteomyelitis or involvement of retrosternal organs and tissues(3).

The mediastinum is conventionally divided into three parts: anterior, middle and posterior. Mediastinitis following cardiac surgery is anterior, unlike ENT, resophageal or dental mediastinitis, which are usually posterior.

It is a dreadful complication, requiring urgent management that combines both a surgical component, based on cleaning and trimming of infected areas, and a medical component, essentially probabilistic antibiotic therapy(4,5).

It is associated with a non-negligible mortality rate, the additional cost of lengthy hospitalisation with significant economic repercussions, and an impact on the socio-professional life of survivors(6,7).

We are interested in the study of postoperative mediastinitis, which is still a very serious complication.

Several studies have focused on the risk factors for developing mediastinitis, with the aim of initiating prevention programmes to limit the incidence of this infection.

Unfortunately, we cannot act on all these factors, some of which are inherent to the characteristics of the population.

This is indeed the problem in cardiac surgery, where the majority of patients have multiple defects.

And despite constant advances in therapeutics and patient management, post-operative mediastinitis remains a formidable complication, unavoidable for some patients (if the benefit/risk ratio is weighed up) but still manageable if properly diagnosed and treated(8).

On the basis of these findings, this study seeks to identify the factors that predict mortality in patients with surgical site infections.

In-depth knowledge of the risk factors and the means of control are the cornerstone of prevention.

The aims of this work were to :
-    Describe the characteristics of patients who have developed this complication.
-    Identify the risk factors for mortality.
-    Determining the mortality rate

2 MATERIALS AND METHODS

I. Type of study

In order to meet the set objectives, a retrospective cross-sectional observational study including patients operated on by vertical median sternotomy was carried out at the HMPIT Cardiothoracic Surgery Department between 1 January 2010 and 31 December 2019.

The study includes a descriptive section on the various clinical, operative and post-operative characteristics of the patients, and an analytical section highlighting the risk factors for mortality and morbidity in this type of procedure.

II.Study population

During this 10-year period, 55 patients developed mediastinitis in our department. The inclusion criteria were:

-    The initial approach: a vertical median sternotomy.
-    The infection is deep (beyond the sternal table).
-    The need for surgical debridement.

III. Definition

Mediastinitis is a deep infection of the operative site following vertical median sternotomy.

As defined by CDC (centres for disease control and prevention)

Elie includes one of the following criteria:

- Isolation of a micro-organism from a mediastinal sample.

-    Evidence of mediastinitis on re-surgery.

-    Chest pain, sternal instability, hyperthermia > 38°C + purulent discharge or positive blood culture.

Table I Definition of mediastinitis according to CDC

Mediastinitis (in adults) must meet at least 1 of the following criteria:

1. Patient has organisms cultured from mediastinal tissue or fluid obtained during a surgical operation or needle aspiration.
2. Patient has evidence of mediastinitis seen during a surgical operation or histopathologic examination.
3. Patient has at least 1 of the following signs or symptoms with no other recognized cause: fever (>38°C), chest pain, or sternal instability.

AND at least 1 of the following:
- purulent discharge from mediastinal area
- organisms cultured from blood or discharge from mediastinal area
- mediastinal widening on radiography

Mediastinitis (in adults) must meet at least 1 of the following criteria!

1.   Patient has organisms cultured from mediastinal tissue or **fluid** obtained during a surgical operation or needle aspiration.

2.   Patient has evidence of mediastinitis seen during a surgical operation or histopathologic examination.

3. Patient has at least I of the following signs or symptoms with no other recognised cause: fever (>38 C), chest pain, or sternal instability.
AND at least I of the following:
*   purulent discharge from mediastinal area
*   organisms cultured from blood or discharge from mediastinal area
*   mediastinal widening on radiography

- BMI: Body Mass Index as defined by the World Health Organisation, it indicates whether the individual is underweight (BMI<18.5), normally built (18.5 = BMI<25), overweight (25 = BMI<30) or obese (BMI=30).

- Euroscore II: European System for Cardiac Operative Risk Evaluation, a score used to assess the risk of cardiac surgery before the operation, and the expected mortality in this type of patient.

- Cardiac dysfunction: a threshold of LVEF <50% and aTAPSE<18 was taken forVD.

IV. Methods

1. Data collection

Data were collected from medical records, operative notes, anaesthesia records and intensive care unit records in the cardiac and thoracic surgery department of HMPIT, using a predefined template (Appendix 1).

V. Static analysis

The data was entered and analysed using SPSS version 23 software.

1. Descriptive analysis

Categorical variables were expressed by their absolute frequencies (numbers) and their relative frequencies (percentages).

Quantitative variables were expressed by their means and standard deviations when their distributions followed the normal distribution, otherwise by their medians and extreme values.

The variables were tested for normality using the Kolmogorov-Smirnov test. All values are expressed as rounded figures.

2. Analytical study

2.1. Univariate analysis

Percentages were compared using Pearson's Chi 2 test if the conditions of application were verified, otherwise using Fisher's exact test. Means were compared using Student's t test for variables following the Normal distribution, otherwise using the Mann Whitney U test.

2.2. Multivariate analysis

For the multivariate analysis of factors independently associated with postoperative mortality, binary logistic regression was used. The Hosmer-Lemeshow test was used to verify the goodness of fit of the model. In all statistical tests, the significance level was set at 0.05.

3. Keyword search

The bibliography was obtained from various scientific sources available on the Internet.

The scientific search browsers used were : PubMed, ReaserchGate, Google Scholar and Science Direct.

The following keywords were used:

Mediastinitis, cardiac surgery, mortality, infection.

4. Ethical considerations

Prior agreement was obtained from the various heads of department included in the study.

I. Plan of the study

We studied the characteristics of patients who developed mediastinitis after cardiac surgery.

A total of 55 patients were included. 17 patients died, and we are going to determine the contribution of mediastinitis to this mortality.

We studied the characteristics of the overall population and then of each group. The groups were compared in terms of pre-, peri- and post-operative data, as well as their statistical differences in univariate analysis. This will be developed in the following paragraphs.

Finally, the multivariate analyses of each criterion will be detailed.

II. Characteristics of the overall population

1. Presurgical data

1.1. Age

The median age was 61, with an average of 60. The extremes ranged from 21 to 83.

Mediane de Cage

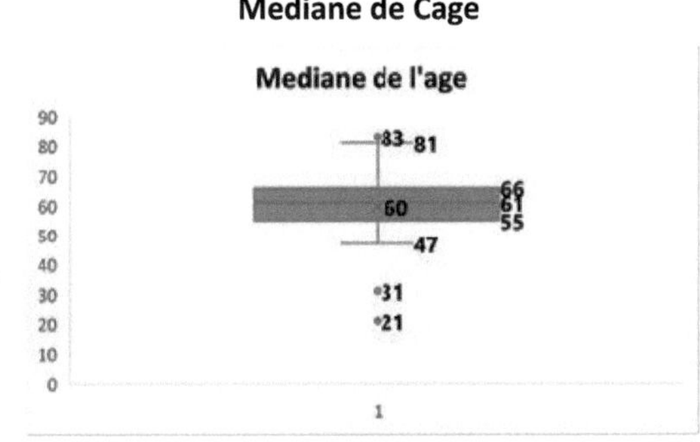

Figure 1 Mean and median of ɼaðe in years.

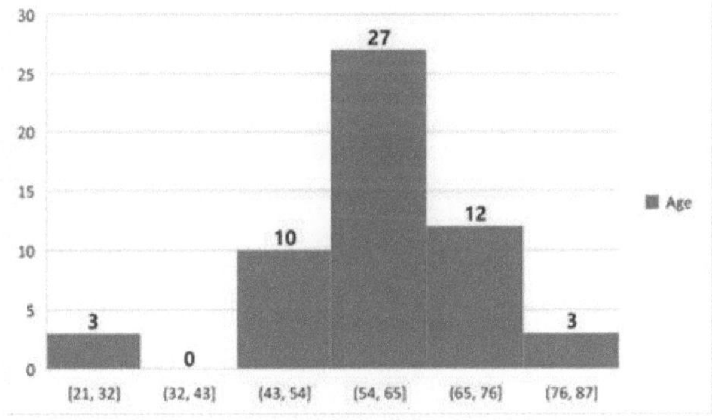

Figure 2 Percentage distribution of the population by age

1.2. Gender

20% (11 patients) were women and 80% (44 patients) were men.

1.3. Overweight and obesity

The median l'IMC was 26 with an average of 31.

27% of patients were overweight, 22% were obese and only one was morbidly obese.

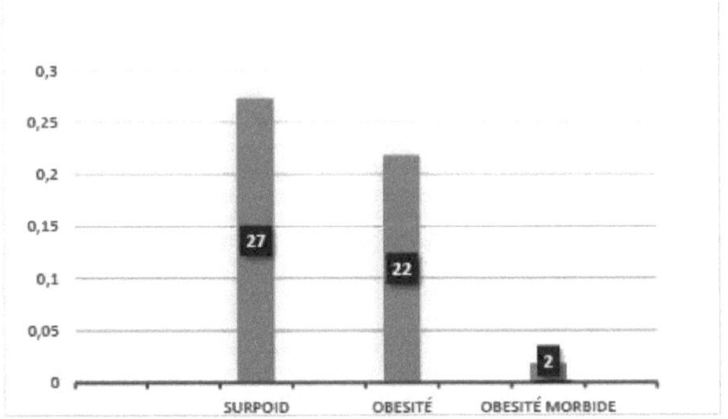

Figure 3 Percentage distribution of the population according to IMC

1.4. Smoking

71% of patients were smokers.

1.5. Comorbidities

84% of patients had at least one comorbidity, dominated by hypertension, diabetes and dyslipidemia.

23% of diabetics were poorly balanced (the median HbAlc was 8, with values ranging from 5 to 12), mostly type II (97%), with an estimated median age of 10 years.

2 patients were on corticosteroids.

All these comorbidities are detailed in the graph below.

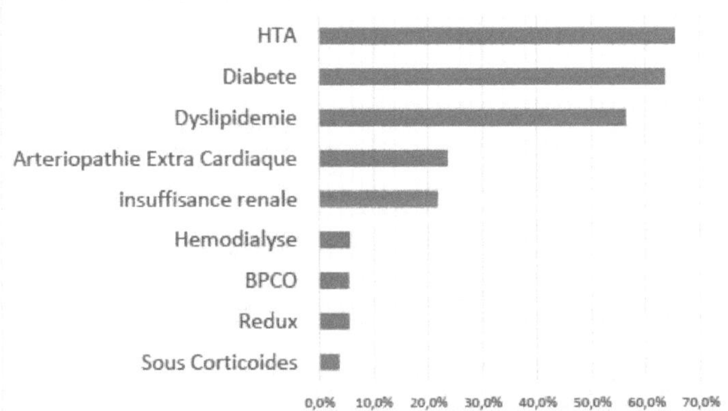

(hypertension, diabetes, dyslipidemia, kidney failure, haemodialysis, COPD, arterial disease).

Figure 4 Percentage distribution of the population by comorbidity

1.6 Euro score II

The average euro score II was 2 and a median of 1 with extremes ranging from 1 a6.

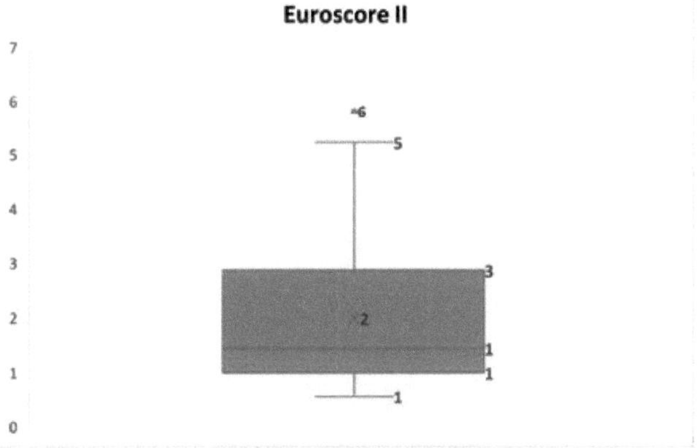

Figure 5 Mean and median Euroscore

1.7 Assessment of cardiac function after bypass :

16 patients had LV dysfunction (29%), 8 patients (20%) had VD dysfunction. The median LVEF was 50% and the mean 48%.

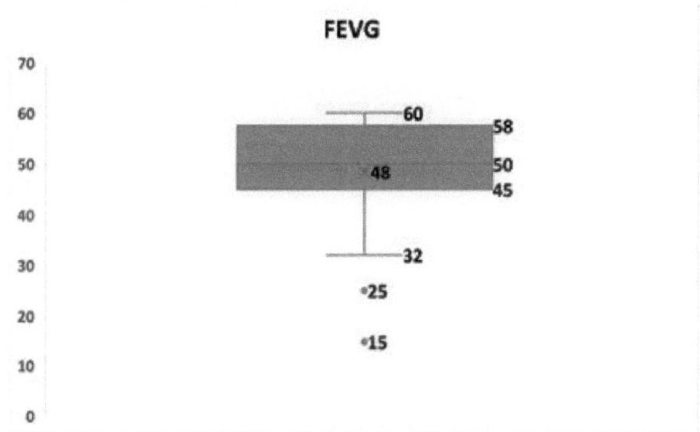

Figure 6 Mean and median LVEF in percent

1.8. Initial intervention data

1.8.1. Type of intervention

73% of the operations were coronary bypasses, 17% valvular bypasses. Two cases of resection of a sub-aortic membrane, one patient operated on for an OG myxoma, one patient operated on for atrial septal defect and one patient operated on for infective endocarditis who benefited from a valve replacement.

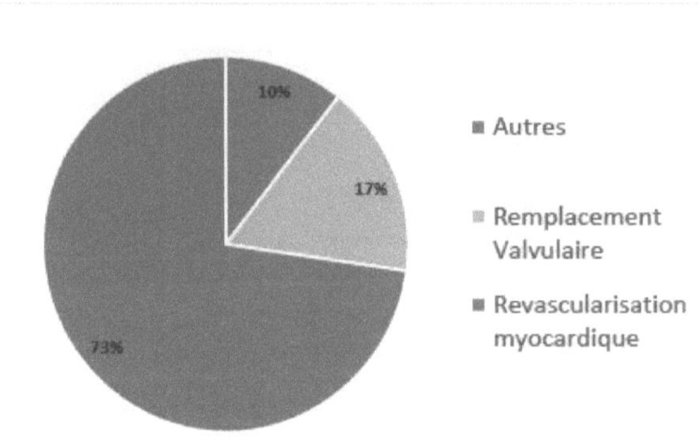

- Other
- Valve replacement
- Myocardial revascularisation

Figure 7 Type of / intervention initiated as a percentage

With regard to myocardial revascularisation, only 14% of patients had recourse to the use of both mammary arteries.

And the median number of revascularised vessels was 3.

It should be noted that 3 patients (5%) were redux patients.

1.8.2. Duration of bypass surgery and aortic clamping

Bypass time was 126 min (median) and aortic clamping 83 min (median).

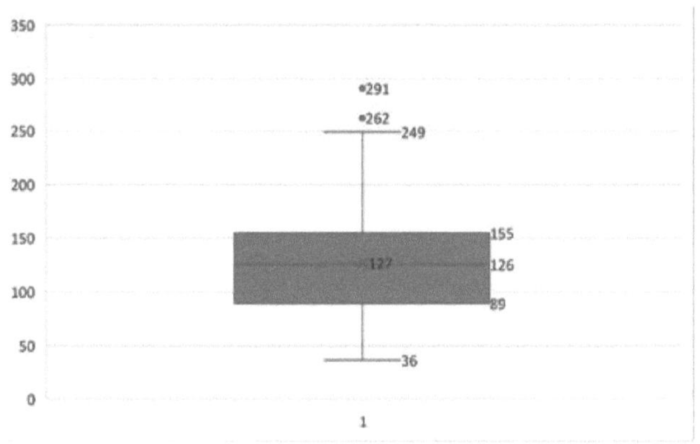

Figure 8 Mean and median CEC time in minutes

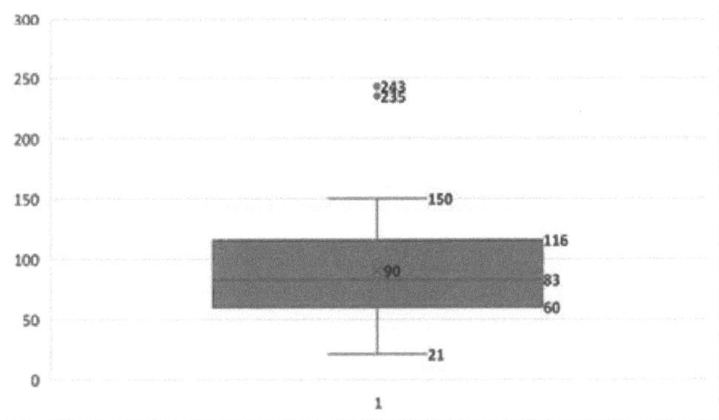

Figure 9 Mean and median aortic clamping time in minutes

1.8.3. Post-ECC complications

The average length of stay in intensive care after bypass surgery was 6 days, with a median of 4 days and extremes ranging from 1 to 23 days.

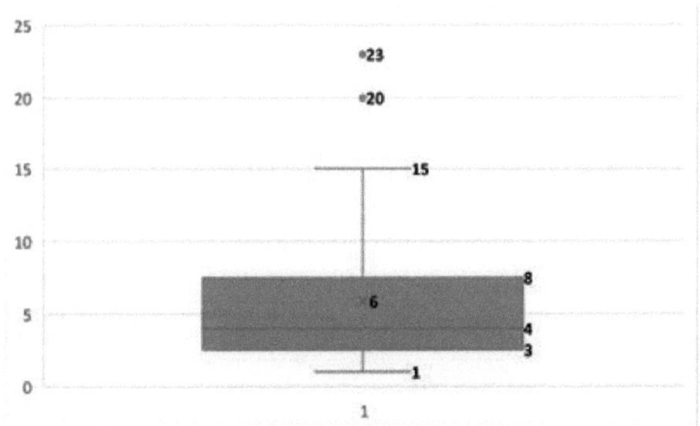

Figure 10 Average and median length of stay in intensive care in days

Post-ECC complications have been subdivided into three main groups: cardiac, septic and other.

10 patients (18%) developed post-CEC cardiac dysfunction, of whom 4 (7%) required cardiac assistance such as ECMO or counter-pulsation balloons.

22 patients (40%) had sepsis, mainly of pulmonary origin (20 patients, 36%), with respiratory distress in 25% (14 patients).

It should be noted that 9 patients required reintubation (16%).

8 patients (14%) required hemodialysis out of the 14 patients (25%) with renal failure.

6 patients (11%) were re-explored for hemostasis.

Other complications are detailed in the chart below.

It should be noted that the initial post-CEC ventilation time was 6 days on average and 36 days on average.

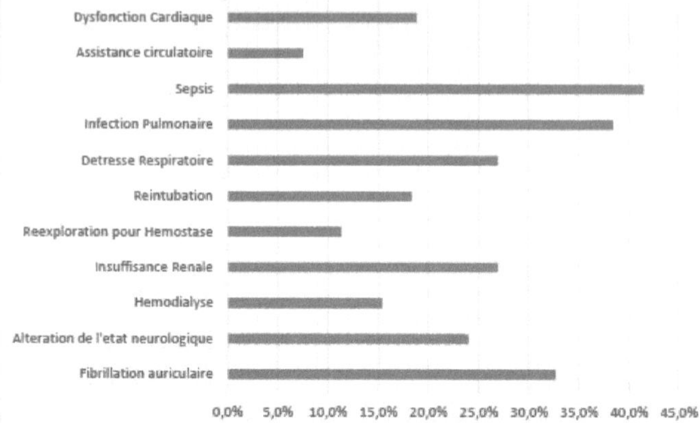

Figure 11 Percentage distribution of the population according to the type of complications developed after bypass surgery

2. Diagnostic elements
2.1. Total population

Delays in treatment in relation to the onset of symptoms are detailed in the table below.

Table II Treatment times for the overall population in days

Population Global	Average	Mediane	Minimum value	Maximum value
Time to onset of symptoms	9	9	1	24
Interval between onset of symptoms and diagnosis	3	1	0	27
Interval between diagnosis and recovery	1	0	0	4

2.2. Patients diagnosed during the stay :

78%, or 43 of the patients, were diagnosed during the same hospitalisation for the first operation.

Patients diagnosed during the same hospital stay were subdivided into two subgroups: those diagnosed in the intensive care unit and those diagnosed on the ward.

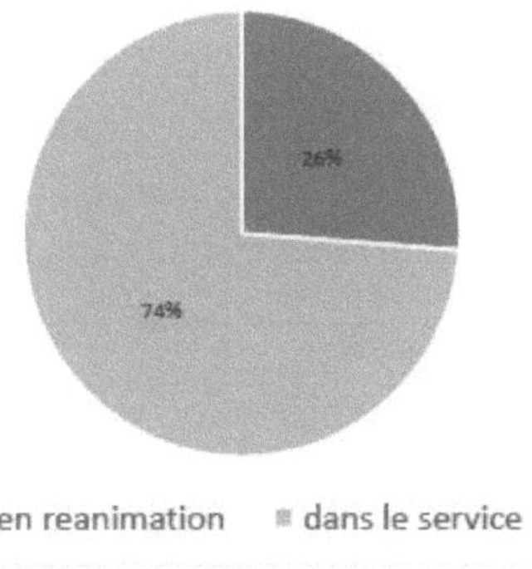

Figure 12 Breakdown of the population by length of stay at the time of diagnosis in percentage

2.3. Patients diagnosed in the intensive care unit versus those diagnosed on the ward

Management times were longer for patients diagnosed in intensive care than for those diagnosed on the ward. Management times are detailed in the table below.

Table III Oë/ai of care for patients 41aдno5йдuë during their stay in days

Diagnosis during your stay	Time to onset of symptoms		Interval between symptomatology and diagnosis		Interval between diagnosis and recovery		Interval between onset of symptoms and recovery	
	Service	Rea	Service	Rea	Servic Rea e		Service	Rea
Average	10	8	23		1	1	3	4
Mediane	9	7	12		0	1	1	3

3. Patients diagnosed after discharge

12 patients (22%) developed symptoms after hospital discharge.

Table IV Oë!a1 management for patients diagnosedë after discharge in days

Diagnosis after discharge	Average	Mediane
Time to onset of symptoms	10	9
Interval between symptomatology and admission	2	1
Interval between Admission and Recovery	1	1

4. Diagnostic elements

With regard to clinical signs, we have concentrated on those presented in the literature: in our series, fever is the most common, with or without associated sternal discharge, sternal instability, local inflammation, loss of skin or chest pain.

The percentages shown in the table below represent the total population.

Table V Clinical warning signs in the general population

Total population	Percentage
Fever	64%
Chest pain	12%
From Serosite	38%
From Pus	31%
Sternal instability	36%
Scar Inflammation	27%
Loss of Cutaneous Substance	10%

We then subdivided the population into three groups according to the time of diagnosis: in intensive care, on the ward or after the initial discharge.

Table VI Clinical signs of patients diagnosed in intensive care

Diagnosis in intensive care	Percentage	
Fever	90%	
Chest pain		0%
From Serosite	10%	
From Pus	20%	
Sternal instability	20%	
Scar Inflammation		0%
Loss of Cutaneous Substance		0%

Table VII Clinical warning signs for patients diagnosed after discharge from hospital

Diagnosis after initial discharge	Percentage
Fever	42%
Chest pain	36%
From Serosite	42%
From Pus	42%
Sternal instability	42%
Scar Inflammation	33%
Loss of Cutaneous Substance	42%

Only 38% of cases were considered urgent, and the diagnosis was based on clinical data in the majority of cases (57%).

It should be noted that 64% of patients diagnosed in intensive care had a thoracic CT scan prior to diagnosis.

At the time of diagnosis, 28% of patients were in a critical condition, as detailed in the graph below.

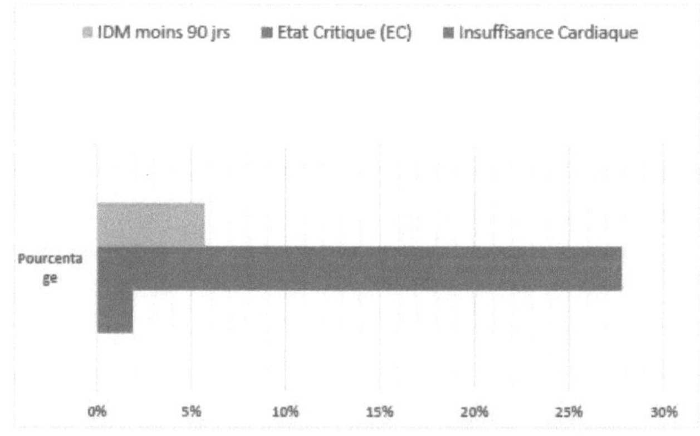

Figure 13 Distribution of the population according to the severity of their condition at the time of diagnosis

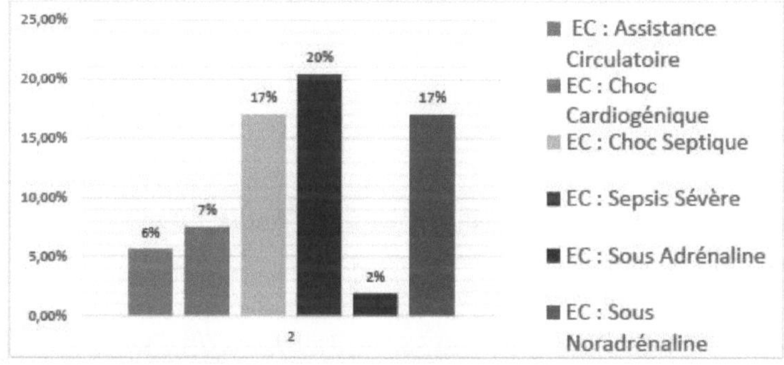

Figure 14 Distribution of the population according to the nature of their critical condition

Of these patients, 20% were already in intensive care.

4.1. Paraclinical diagnostic elements

4.1.1. Biological elements

Bases on CRP, leukocytes, procalcitonin if available and preoperative haemoglobin are detailed in the table below.

Table VIII The biological ë1ëmeM$ before the takeover.

Pre-takeover	Average	Mediane	Minimum	Maximum
Hemoglobin	9	8	7	14
Leukocyte	16	15	7	39
CRP	221	213	26	628
PCT	14	1	0	200

4.1.2. Pre-operative bacteriological data

Whenever possible (except in cases of extreme urgency), a series of blood cultures and a local sample from the operating site were taken.

Only 12 samples were positive, the majority identifying a staphylococcus (aureus, coagulase negative, Methi S, Methi R).

4.1.3. Pre-resumption antibiotic therapy

70% of patients underwent probabilistic antibiotic treatment prior to surgery for suspected mediastinitis.

The median duration of antibiotic treatment is estimated at 3 days and the average at

5 days for the overall population.

This period is longer for those diagnosed in intensive care than for those diagnosed in the preoperative unit.

Table IX Duration of antibiotic treatment before resumption

Duration of TBA	Mean	Median	Minimum	Maximum
In intensive care	7	5	4	11
In department	5	2	1	18

Most of the antibiotics taken were for infectious pneumonia following bypass surgery, which was a cause of diagnostic delay.

5. Intraoperative data

Surgical treatment was based on exploration of the wound, debridement of devitalized and necrotic tissue, and removal of the sternal sutures.

Intraoperative sampling was systematic.

All patients underwent closure during the same operation.

No patient required reconstruction using muscle flaps or VACtherapy (vacuum-assisted closure).

The difference was in the sealing technique (steel wire) and the choice of suction system.

5.1. Closing techniques

In comparing the techniques for closing the sternum, we opted for three methods: simple interrupted steel wires combined in some cases with lateral support wires (modified Robicsek technique) (45%), simple and "X" wires (32%).

The median number of steel wires applied during surgical closure of the sternum was 6 and 8, if we include the lateral wires used.

5.2. Surgical drainage

Routine drainage with Redivac continuous suction (94% of cases), combined in some cases with No. 30-32 French chest tubes, was performed in all patients for at least 15 days.

6. Post-operative data

6.1. Post-operative complications

6.1.1. Stay in intensive care

58% of patients required an ICU stay, as detailed in the table below.

Table X Length of stay in post-recovery intensive care in days

Length of stay in intensive care recovery	Mean	Median	Minimum	Maximum
	9	3	1	78

6.1.2. Immediate post-recovery complications

None of the patients required hemodynamic support or immediate post-operative recovery.

The other complications are detailed below.

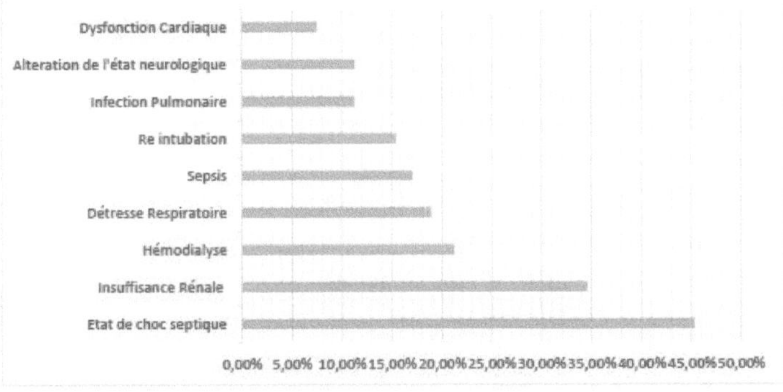

Figure 15 Breakdown of the population by type of post-recovery complications (%)

The majority of patients admitted to intensive care developed septic shock with impaired renal function.

Followed by respiratory distress requiring intubation in 44% of cases. And in this table we have detailed the complications concerning patients diagnosed in intensive care.

Table XI Post-recovery complications in patients diagnosed in the intensive care unit

	Percentage
Re intubation	44%
Lung infection	44%
Respiratory distress	67%
Cardiac dysfunction	11%
Alteration of the neurological state	22%
Septic shock	89%
Sepsis	22%

Renal insufficiency	78%
Hemodialysis	44%

6.1.3. Post-operative biological data

CRP levels, haemoglobin and the need for transfusion were studied.

41 patients required an intraoperative or postoperative transfusion, as detailed in this table.

Table XII Post-operative biological data

	Average	Mediane	Minimum	Maximum
Number of red blood cells transfuse	1	1	0	5
Hemoglobin (minimum) in g/dl	9	9	5	12
CRP (maximum)	212	185	30	475

6.1.4. Post-operative microbiological data

56% of patients had a positive local intraoperative sample.

The median duration of in-hospital antibiotic treatment was estimated at 21 days, followed by 3 weeks of oral therapy on discharge.

6.1.5. Duration of thoracic drainage

Thoracic drainage was maintained for an average of 12 days, with a median of 10 days and extremes of 3 and 42 days.

6.1.6. Post-operative complications: Recurrence of infection

These included persistent infection, fistulisation of the skin, discharge (pus or serositis), loss of skin tissue and recurrence of mediastinitis. It should be noted that four repeat cases were related to recurrence of mediastinitis and only one to hemostasis.

For superficial wall infections, local treatment with colloid dressings has produced satisfactory results.

Table XIII Local post-operative complications

Type of complication	Percentage
Recurrence of Mediastinitis	9%
Surgical revision	11%
Persistence of ('Infection	26%
Fistulisation of the skin	2%
Flow	22%
Loss of skin substance	11%

6.1.7. Post-resumption stay

Table XIV Postoperative 5ë]ouz durations in days.

	Average	Mediane	Standard deviation	Minimum	Maximum
Length of stay in intensive care	6	3	15	1	78
Duration of post-operative stay	21	19	14	1	78
Total length of stay	38	35	18	3	97

7. Deaths

17 patients (31%) died postoperatively, including 5 (9%) from septic shock.

II. Comparison of the two groups: survivors versus decedents: univariate study

1. Factors predictive of pre-operative mortality

Univariate analysis showed that the following variables were predictive of peroperative mortality:

DV dysfunction, LV function, length of stay in intensive care unit post-CEC, need for circulatory assistance, development of cardiac dysfunction, alteration in neurological status, recourse to re-intubation, sepsis, atrial fibrillation and hemodialysis.

Also diagnosis during a stay in intensive care, serositis tissue, use of

noradrenaline, septic shock, local sampling before recovery.

Table XV Univariate study of demographic data and antecedents in the overall population predictive of mortality

Ооппёез Dëmographic and ап1ёсёдеп1з population ёtudiёe				Study 11пМапё
	Total population	Population dëcëdëe	Surviving population	OR Chi-square test [Minimum- Maximum]
	Number Percentage	Number Percentage	Number Percentage	
Right ventricular dysfunction	820%	562%	39%	nnn "16,11 [2.5- **0,001** ' ' rl 103.5

Table XVI Univariate study of preoperative data predictive of mortality

Ооппёез prë opёra1o!re population ё1ид!ёе						
	Total population		Population dëcëdëe		Surviving population		Study 11пК/апё
	Average	Mëdiane	Average	Mëdiane	Average	Mëdiane	
LVEF (%)	48	50	36	38	51	53	**0.001**

Table XVII Univariate study of preoperative factors predictive of mortality in the initial operation

	Oоппёез prё opёra1o!re population ёtudiёe					Study итуапё
	Total population		Population dёcёdёe		Surviving population	
	Average	Mёdian	Average	Mёdian	Average	Mёdiane
Онгёе зё]оиг post ECC resuscitation.	64		97		4	3	**0,003**

Table XVIII Univariate study of post-ECC complications predictive of mortality

	Oоппёез prё opёra1o!re population ёtudiёe					Study 11пMапё	
Post CEC complication	Total population		Population dёcёdёe		Surviving population		
	Total workforce	Percentage	Workforce	Percentage	Workforce	Percentage	Test Chi-square 2	OR [Minimum - Maximum]
Circulatory assistance	4	7%	4	23%	0	0%	**0,002**	3,77 [2,37-6]
Cardiac dysfunction	10	19%	6	35%	4	11%	**0,036**	4,36 [1,04-18,4]
VD dysfunction	8	20%	5	62%	3	9%	**0,001**	16,11 [2,51-103,55]
Alteration of neurological condition	12	24%	7	47%	5	14%	**0,014**	5,25 [1,31-21,03]
Re intubation	9	18%	5	38%	4	11%	**0,029**	5 [1,09-23]
Sepsis	22	41%	11	65%	11	31%	**0,019**	4,17 [1,23-14,14]
Atrial fibrillation	17	33%	10	62%	7	19%	**0,002**	6,9 [1,88-25,49]
f^modialysis	8	15%	5	31%	3	8%	**0,035**	5 [1,02-24,41]

Table XIX Univariate study of factors predictive of mortality according to place of diagnosis

		Oоппёез prё opёra1o!re population ёtudiёe			Surviving population	Study 11пMапё	
		Total population	Population dёcёdёe				
Diagnosis of	Mediastinitis	Total effect	Percentage	Number Percentage	Number Percentage	Test Chi-square 2	OR [Min - Max]
During your stay	In intensive care	11	26%	857%	311%	**0,001**	11,11 [2,25-54,94]
	In the department	31	74%	643%	2589%	****	

Table XX Univariate study of warning signs predictive of mortality

	Oоппёез prё opёra1o!re population ё1ид!ёе Study 11пMапё				
Table Clinic	Total population	Population dёcёdёe	Surviving population	Chi 2 test	OR [Minimum - Maximum]

	Total Percentage	Number Percentage Number Percentage			
	Total Percentage	Number Percentage	Number Percentage		
Issue зёгозкё	2038%	17%	1951%	**0,003**	0,067 [0,008-0,57]

Table XXI Univariate study of clinical features at the time of diagnosis predictive of mortality

Ооппёез прё opёra1o!re population ё1ид!ёе Study 11пК/апё

Overall population Population dёcёdёe Surviving population QD

Clinical condition	Total workforce	Percentage	Workforce	Percentage	Workforce	Percentage	Test Chi-square 2	[Minimum - Maximum]
Heart failure	1	2%	1	7%	0	0%	**0,108** **	
IDM minus 90	3	6%	3	20%	0	0%	**0,005** **	
Critical State	15	28%	10	62%	5	13%	**0**	11 [2,76-43,8]
Assistance Circulatory	3	6%	3	19%	0	0%	**0,006** **	
Shock Cardiogёnique	4	7%	4	27%	0	0%	**0,001** **	
Septic shock	9	17%	6	40%	3	8%	**0,005**	7,78 [1,62-37,3]
"i-Sepsis 5ёyёre	11	20%	8	50%	3	8%	**0**	11,67 [2,52-54,05]
Under Adrenaline	1	1%	1	7%	0	0%	**0,11** **	
Under Noradrenaline	9	17%	6	40%	3	8%	**0,005**	7,78 [1,62-37,3]

Table XXII Univariate study of diagnostic factors predictive of mortality

	Ооппёез prё opёra1o!re population ё1ид!ёе						Study 11пМапё
Overall population Population dёcёdёe Surviving population						OR [Minimum Maximum]	
DiagnosticTest							
	Number	Percentage	Number	Percentage	Number	Percentage	Chi-square 2
Levy							
Local Prё Takeover	29	59%	3	23%	26	72%	**0,002** [0,03-0,51]

Table XXIII Univariate study of diagnostic factors predictive of mortality

Ооπёез Pre	Ооппёез prё opёra1o!re population ёtudiёe						Study
	Total population		Population dёcёdёe		Surviving population		U пп/апё
Takeover	Average	Mёdian	Average	Mёdian	Average	Mёdian	
CRP (Max)	221213		289279		193175		**0,01**

2. Factors predictive of intra- and post-operative mortality

Postoperative resuscitation, reintubation, respiratory distress, septic shock, the development of renal failure and recourse to hemodialysis were retained in the univariate study as predictive factors of postoperative mortality.

Recurrence of mediastinitis, persistent infection and discharge were also found to be predictive of post-operative mortality.

Table XXIV Univariate study of postoperative data predictive of mortality

	Post-operative data for the population studied					Univarie study	
	Total population		Deceased population		Surviving population	Test Chi-square 2	OR [Minimum Maximum]
Post Opёra1oие	Total	Percentage	Number	Percentage	Number Percentage		
Stay in resuscitation	3158%		1493%		1745%	0,001	17,29 [2,06-145,11]

Table XXV Univariate study of postoperative complications predictive of mortality

Post Recovery Complication	Donr^es post opёra1o!re population ё1ид!ёе						Study 11п1уапё
	Total population		Population dёcёdёe		Surviving population	Test Chi-square 2	OR [Minimum - Maximum]
	Total effect	Percentage	Effect if	Percentage	Workforce Percentage		
Re exploration	0	0%	0	0%	0	0%	**0,022** 5,67 [1,15-27,94]
Assistance	0	0%	0	0%	0	0%	**0,027** 6,55 [1,05-40,67]
Re intubation	8	15%	5	33%	3	8%	**0,013** 5,67 [1,31-24,47]
Oё1re$5e Respiratory	10	19%	6	40%	4	10%	**0,001** 18,5 [1,94-176,9]
Cardiac dysfunction	4	7%	2	13%	2	5%	**0** 39,2 [4,55-337,68]
Septic shock	24	45%	14	93%	10	26%	**0,014** 4,67 [1,3-16,74]
Insufficiency rёna1e	18	35%	9	60%	9	24%	**0,022** 5,67 [1,15-27,94]

I^modialysis	11	21%	5	33%	6	16%	**0,027**	6,55 [1,05-40,67]

Table XXVI Univariate study of the development of sepsis as a predictor of mortality

Oопёез population ëtudiëe	Study ип1уапё		
	Chi 2 test	OR	Minimum - Maximum
5ерьсёт!е Post CEC	**0,035**	3,53	1,07 -11,7
5ерьсёт!е Admission	**0**	17,33	4,19 - 71,7
5ерьсёт!е Post Reprise	**0,001**	10,31	2,06 -1,58
5ерьсёт!е	**0,001**	**	**

Table XXVII Univariate study of intraoperative and postoperative data predictive of mortality

Donr^es per et post opёra1o!re de la population ё1ид!ёе

Oопёез per et post opёra1o!re	Total population		Population dёcёdёе		Surviving population		Study U пп/апё
	Average	Mёdiane	Average	Mёdiane	Average	Mёdiane	
Number of packed red blood cells	1,12	1,00	2,10	2,00	0,81	0,00	**0,04**
CRP	211,87	185,50	297,18	316,00	185,06	174,00	**0,009**

Table XXVIII Univariate study of postoperative factors predictive of mortality

Oоппёез post opёra1o!re population   ёtudiёeEtude Univanё

Post-Takeover Suites	Total population		Population dёcёdёе		Surviving population		Test Chi-square 2	OR [Minimum - Maximum]
	Total workforce	Percentage	Workforce	Percentage	Workforce	Percentage		
Pё<^|ye Mёdiastinitis	4	9%	3	37%	1	3%	**0,001**	22,2 [1,92-256,82]
Surgical revision	5	11%	4	50%	1	2%	**0**	37 [3,28-416,92]
Persistence Infection	12	26%	5	62%	7	18%	**0,01**	7,38 [1,42-38,42]
Flow перси1апё	10	22%	5	62%	5	13%	**0,002**	11 [1,98-60,99]

III. Risk factors: multivariate study

Age over 60 and admission in critical condition were identified as independent predictors of mortality.

While an initial post-CEC ventilation time of more than 4 hours and a LVEF >50% have been identified as independent protective factors for mortality.

Table XXIX: Multivariate study of factors predictive of mortality

Variables	Meaning	OR		IC
Age >60	**0,036**	61,913	1,308	2930,032
Юигёе initial post-CEC ventilation >4 hours	**0,033**	0,010	0,000	0,687
Critical ё1а1 admission	**0,021**	38,327	1,752	838,540
FEVG conзeryё	**0,017**	0,068	0,008	0,614

4 DISCUSSION

The sternotomy is still considered the reference incision for cardiac surgery, despite the revolution in minimally invasive and robotic surgery(9).

It offers excellent exposure and allows visual and manual control of the entire operating field(IO).

And that despite the management of risk factors and the precautions taken, the occurrence of infection is inextricably linked to certain immutable characteristics(2).

The explanation for these differences is multifactorial: the definitions of infection differ from one author to another. There are two definitions of mediastinitis following cardiac surgery. A restrictive definition is based on the need for repeat surgery with positive culture of mediastinal samples or with a macroscopic appearance of mediastinitis.

It can be used to identify the most serious patients, but may miss early-onset mediastinitis. The other, broader definition is essentially based on the concept of deep mediastinal surgical site infection proposed by the US Centers for Disease Control and Prevention (CDC)(4,II). In general, studies based on the restrictive definition have reported a lower incidence of mediastinitis than studies using a CDC-type definition(4,12).

The available French series show a rate of mediastinitis in the order of 2 to 3% according to the CDC definition(5,13), and a rate of 1 to 1.5% when the infection is defined by the repeat operation.

As defined by the CDC(5), mediastinitis remains a serious infectious complication of cardiac surgery with a high mortality rate(8).

Antibiotic therapy and surgical debridement of infected tissue are the cornerstones of treatment. The timing of surgery is crucial, as early as possible to avoid the spread of infection(14).

Properly managed, the damage to survival, quality of life and socio-economic status is always significant(15).

Elie has a variable incidence and a non-negligible mortality rate ranging from 10% to 35% and 40% in some series (2,16) and 30.9% in our population.

However, the incidences reported in the literature vary widely, from 0.25% to 6.5%.

In our series, the population was predominantly of 3eme age, with a median of 61 years, multi-tare, 84% had at least one comorbidity, with a male predominance of 80%.

Dominated by hypertension (65.5%), diabetes (63.6%), and dyslipidemia (56.4%).

The initial surgical procedure was coronary bypass in 73% of cases, and most patients were diagnosed during the same hospital stay (78%), whether in intensive care or on the ward (74%).

The clinical presentation was dominated by fever (64%), with 15 patients (28%) in a critical condition at diagnosis.

Chest CT scans were used for diagnosis in 43% of patients, mainly when the clinical picture was poor.

In fact, fever was the only sign present in 9 patients, and these are usually the patients diagnosed in intensive care.

And despite the large number of bacteriological samples taken, only 55% were positive, mostly for staphylococcus.

Post-operative septic shock was the most serious complication, accounting for 45% of cases and 5 deaths.

Given the critical condition of the patients, the other deaths were related to cardiac or septic failure with a pulmonary origin.

These data show us how difficult it is to manage mediastinitis, despite the fact that it is well codified, and the need for polyvalent treatment(2).

I. Descriptive analysis

1. Pre-operational data

1.1. Demographic data

1.1.1. Age

With a mean age of 59 and a median age of 61, our population is younger than most of the series (17-19) (which defines age over 70 as a risk factor). This is comparable to that described previously in Tunisia by Kallel et al, Ouerchefani et al(12,20).

In fact, this is consistent with the fact that some series studying sternal healing have shown that age over 45 is an independent risk factor for delayed sternal healing, itself an important prognostic factor in the development of mediastinitis(21).

This age difference can be explained by the fact that the advent and development of interventional cardiology means that patients proposed for surgery are older(15) with more comorbidities, particularly for coronary surgery or combined surgery, techniques which are more developed in the West than in Tunisia(16,22).

1.1.2. Type

80% of the patients included in our study were men, as were the two Tunisian series(12,20). The predominance of women(23-27) or men(7,15,17,28) differs according to the series and the characteristics of each population.

An increased risk in women is due, according to some authors, to the difference in fat distribution and a more deficient peripheral circulation in women than in men

(23).

Others suggest that the increased infero-lateral tension exerted by the size of the breasts on the sternotomy wound contributes to wound dehiscence and subsequent infection(26,27).

1.1.3. BMI

Only 20% of our population were of normal build. Obesity as a risk factor for mediastinitis has been widely studied(17,19,25,26,28,29), with a prevalence comparable to our series. Several mechanisms are involved, including the pharmacokinetics and pharmacodynamics of drugs, which are difficult to estimate and reduce the bioavailability of drugs, especially antibiotics. There is also an increase in post-operative mechanical loads and a decrease in the vascularisation of adipose tissue, which can adversely affect wound healing(23,26,30-32).

1.1.4. Tobacco

The majority of our patients were smokers, with a percentage of 71%. This percentage is clearly higher than that described in the literature(15,17).

We have not found enough studies reporting the direct impact of smoking on the genesis of mediastinitis.

However, some authors suggest that tobacco weakens the immune system and alters tissue microcirculation, thereby delaying wound healing. It may also contribute to the genesis of infection by altering the nasopharyngeal flora and accentuating coughing (l,17,33,34).

1.2. Antecedents

Dominated by hypertension, diabetes and dyslipidemia in our series.

Hypertension and dyslipidemia have been reported in the literature, but are not known to be factors implicated in the direct genesis of infection(17,35). However, they are important cardiovascular risk factors that should be considered in all patients.

On the other hand, Ali U, et al(36) mentioned in their study the importance of hypercholesterolemia as a protective factor by modelling the inflammatory reaction.

20% of our population have peripheral vascular network damage comparable to that found by Perrault et al(37) and M.G.Fakih et al(38). This damage is an important factor in the operability assessment: vascular damage to the supra-aortic trunks and post-operative neurological prognosis.

Obliterative arteriopathy of the lower limbs can also be treated if peripheral circulatory assistance is required.

1.2.1. Diabetes

Diabetes has been shown to be one of the most important predictors of mediastinitis, present in the majority of series, multiplying the risk of infection with a prevalence comparable to that in our population(12,17,20,37).

Chronic hyperglycaemia has harmful consequences for the immune system, interfering with sternal healing. Furthermore, vascular damage in the early stages of the disease contributes to hypoxia and ischaemia of local tissues(24,26,39).

The American Diabetes Society recommends a preoperative HbAlc of <7% whenever possible. The recommended upper limit of glycemia is 1.8g/dl during the pre-, per- and post-operative period, and continuous insulin infusions should be used if necessary(l,23,34).

Diabetes is a major topic of debate in terms of myocardial revascularisation, especially arterial revascularisation. Some authors have demonstrated that the inflammatory process generated by infection alters graft quality and long-term survival(28,39,40).

1.2.2. Renal insufficiency

Renal failure is a powerful and independent factor in the occurrence of infection(17,24,37,41).

22% of our patients had altered renal function and only 3 patients (6%) had chronic hemodialysis. Low prevalence was reported in the majority of series, with varying degrees of severity.

A reduced glomerular filtration rate is associated with an increased risk of surgical site infection. Biancari et al showed that an estimated glomerular filtration rate of less than 60 ml/min/1.73 m2 was associated with an almost two-fold increased risk of surgical site infection (24,41).

The immune dysregulation caused by uremia and the poor general condition of renal failure patients may also explain this susceptibility to surgical site infection(24,41).

Finally, with an increased risk of intraoperative bleeding, renal failure may be indirectly associated with postoperative infection(24,41).

1.2.3. COPD and corticosteroid therapy

The prevalence of patients with COPD was very low in our population, 6% or 3 patients. This prevalence is low compared with that found in the literature (17,18,28,42).

This low prevalence may be due to the fact that the majority of COPD patients are often unrecognised and not followed up(12,20).

Multiplying the risk by 2.5, Abdelnoor et al and Phoon et al(18,43) reported two main factors: constant bacterial colonisation in COPD patients and coughing, which causes sternal instability.

1.2.4. Cardiac function

Bi-ventricular function in our series was satisfactory in most patients.

This average is equivalent to the references found for an average LVEF of between 50 and 55%.

The series defines patients with left ventricular dysfunction (<45%) as likely to develop a surgical site infection(23,25,36).

We have not found any studies detailing right heart dysfunction as a single entity, but rather either overall heart dysfunction or left heart dysfunction.

Cardiac dysfunction has a major impact in the post-operative period: prolonged stay in intensive care, use of high doses of catecholamines, low cardiac output, etc., all of which favour alteration of tissue perfusion and accentuate vasoconstriction, thus contributing to the genesis of infection and constituting a major factor in morbidity and mortality(25).

1.3. Data from the first operation

1.3.1. Nature of the initial operation

Coronary artery bypass grafting was the most commonly performed surgery, with a percentage of 73%. This prevalence is comparable to that found in the literature studied(15,28,39,44-47) and that of kallel et al(12).

In a systematic review of the Japanese literature, Hirahara et al(47) noted a significant regression in the number of coronary bypass operations in favour of angioplasty, with more combined surgeries for younger subjects. However, coronary bypass surgery remains associated with an increased risk of infection.

Although only 14% of our patients benefited from bi-mammary revascularisation, shown to be an important risk factor offering the patient a better quality of life in the long term, this rate is very low compared with that described by the majority of series, but comparable with that published by kallel et al(12), given the habits of our department.

Mammary artery harvesting techniques have been widely studied in the literature, with skeleton versus pedicle harvesting, and radial artery harvesting as an alternative, especially in obese and diabetic patients, in order to preserve sternal vascularisation as much as possible(43-46).

The number of revascularised vessels does not appear to be a determining factor, although it does appear to play a role in prolonging bypass time.

Patients who have undergone valve replacement alone or a combined revascularisation procedure, or who have developed infective endocarditis, are more likely to have had complicated operative sequelae requiring prolonged stays in intensive care, circulatory assistance, high doses of catecholamines, low cardiac output, etc., an environment that favours the genesis of infection, as described above(4).

1.3.2. Extracorporeal circulation

All patients were operated on under extracorporeal circulation, with arterial cannulation at the foot of the brachio-cephalic arterial trunk and a cannula at the level of the right atrium, or bi-cave cannulation with a left offload placed through the right superior pulmonary vein.

Myocardial protection was provided by a solution of warm cardioplegia at normothermia.

The duration of extracorporeal circulation is estimated at 125 min and 83 min for the duration of aortic clamping.

This can be explained by the complexity of certain surgical procedures, the number of vessels to be revascularised, and even more so in the case of combined or redux surgery.

These times differ considerably between the series, with an aortic clamping time of 48 min and a bypass time of 81 min for Ali U, et al(36) compared with 84 min of aortic clamping and 112 min of bypass for Chan et al(17).

1.3.3. Complications following extracorporeal circulation

The post-operative consequences of the CEC described in our series can be subdivided into two main groups: surgical and medical. These in turn are subdivided into: cardiac, neurological, pulmonary, metabolic and infectious.

Surgical re-exploration, mainly for hemostasis, described by J.C.Y. Lu et al(48) and Oliveira et al(49), is less frequent than that found in our series.

Elie multiplies the risk by 3 or even 6 according to certain authors(26,29,48), by the re-exposure of the mediastinum to the environment thus increasing the risk of contamination of the wound as well as the asepsis conditions which are sometimes deficient given the urgent nature of the procedure and the conditions of the recovery.

The need for massive transfusions, (alteration of the hemodynamic state, recourse to catecholamines. Each complication only gives rise to others, thereby increasing the risk of infection.

The need for cardiac assistance differs in the series depending on the population studied, but the majority of authors identify as independent factors associated complications such as bleeding, ischaemia, hypoperfusion, etc(9,36,37).

Another equally important entity to identify is respiratory and infectious damage, indicating in some cases prolonged intubation or reintubation following respiratory distress, our results being comparable with those of certain series(9,18,38,48).

In their study, Fu et al reported that prolonged positive pressure ventilation exerts a stress effect on the chest wall, contributing to micro-movements which promote sternal instability(9).

Kallel et al(12) in their series only mentioned early surgical revision and transfusion as two independent risk factors. It should be noted that 28% of their population required prolonged intubation.

Regardless of the type of complication described, it significantly lengthens the length of stay in intensive care and worsens the patient's prognosis, thus creating a favourable environment for the onset of mediastinal infection(36). This creates a potential rather than an additive effect.

1.4. Diagnosis

1.4.1. Time and circumstances of care

We divided our population into two groups: those diagnosed during the same hospital stay and those diagnosed after discharge from hospital.

Very little has been written about this in the literature.

The majority of series have focused on the time to onset of the first symptom, estimated at 9 days in our series when the diagnosis was made during the same hospitalisation and 16 days if made after the initial discharge, 15 days for Kallel et al(12), between 10 and 15 days in other series(7,17,50) with extremes ranging from 4 days to 45 days.

In fact, patients are generally discharged, barring complications, at 9-10 days post-operatively. As a result, for patients diagnosed in the department, the symptomatology was so precocious, reflecting either the severity of the infectious process, or the fragility of the terrain, or both.

The second important factor is the time taken to treat the disease, i.e. the time between the onset of symptoms and diagnosis.

A median of one day for our series and an average of 3 days with extremes ranging from 0 to 27 days. This result is consistent with that found in the literature, which estimates an average of 3 to 4 days (17,38,50).

This delay reflects the difficulty of diagnosis. If we look at the group of patients diagnosed in intensive care, this time is estimated to be 3 days on average, with a median of 2 days, whereas it is one day for those diagnosed during their stay in the department, with wider extremes. It is therefore more difficult to establish the diagnosis in intensive care, given the combination of a variety of complications, which sometimes results in the main diagnosis being overlooked.

Of the 11 patients admitted to intensive care, 3 were on circulatory support, 7 had pulmonary infections progressing to respiratory depression, 5 had cardiac dysfunction requiring catecholamines and 5 had an altered neurological state.

The poor clinical picture for these patients, as we shall y detail later, was mainly one of prolonged unexplained fever, leading to the development of septic shock, in patients who were already on ATBs (9 patients).

deterioration of the condition, despite optimal treatment, draws attention to other associated pathologies or other diagnostic points of interest, including mediastinitis.

Similarly, the use of imaging and the problem of patients who are sometimes difficult to transport also lengthens this time.

This waiting period would have a serious impact on patients whose condition is not always favourable.

And even if the diagnosis is made, there is still an extra day before the operation is resumed, as opposed to resumption on the same day if the diagnosis was made on the ward.

This is because some patients require special preparation.

78.2% of patients were diagnosed during the same hospital stay, including 26.2% in intensive care.

The estimated length of stay in intensive care after bypass surgery was 4 days. Dubert et al(51) demonstrated in a large cohort of 160 patients that a stay in intensive care, the longer the stay, was associated with a risk (*4.8) of developing a more severe form associated with bacteremia.

Ma and An(ll), in their study of 170 cases, subdivided into three groups according to the onset of symptoms, showed that patients with early mediastinitis had longer stays in intensive care units and more complicated initial operative sequelae.

This is consistent with the findings of Fakih et al(38) where the majority of patients were diagnosed after hospital discharge (63.2%). They had a shorter length of stay in hospital post-CEC and a shorter length of stay in intensive care units post-CEC. This resembles the profiles of our patients who initially had a simple postoperative course and were diagnosed after discharge.

1.4.2. Clinical picture

Early recognition and diagnosis of sternal complications is imperative to ensure rapid management to halt the inflammatory process and its consequences.

Early treatment is a decisive factor in preventing even greater damage(SI).

This leads us to focus on the evocative warning signs.

Dominated by sternal discharge (from pus or serositis) in 69% of cases. Fever followed in 64% of cases in our population. These two signs are the two most common warning signs described in the literature (7,17,26,52).

Kallel et al(12) reported that sternal discharge and scar inflammation were the two most common features.

Sternal discharge is the most prominent clinical sign in the majority of studies(ll,50,51).

Other clinical signs such as fever, chest pain, sternal instability and inflammation of the scar differ according to the population studied.

Under no circumstances should sternal stability preclude diagnosis. Sternal instability, although an important indicator of the depth of involvement, is not as frequently present(ll,50,51). Particular attention should be paid to patients undergoing intensive care, 90% of whose clinical picture consists of persistent or recurrent fever in patients who are already receiving ATBs (mainly for a nosocomial infection originating in the lungs).

1.4.3 Clinical status at diagnosis and degree of urgency

28% of our patients were in critical condition at the time of admission, 73% of whom were already in intensive care for post-CEC complications as detailed above.

In terms of sepsis, 20% were in severe sepsis and 17% in septic shock.

4 patients were transferred to intensive care at the time of diagnosis for severe sepsis, one of whom had already been discharged from hospital.

The severity of the infectious process in patients who are already in a precarious condition only increases morbidity and mortality, indicating the need for urgent surgical debridement in order to break the vicious circle of infection(17,47). In fact, 38.5% of patients required urgent reintervention on the same day.

The literature does not contain any series detailing these points.

1.4.4. Pre-operative microbiological elements

82% of patients had blood cultures taken and 59% had a local preoperative sample taken within the limits of possibility. Of these samples, only 12 were positive, identifying the different subtypes of staphylococcus in 83% of cases. The positivity rate of the samples was significantly lower than that described in the literature, which is generally higher than 60%(4,15,17,37,50,51).

In 70% of cases, antibiotic therapy was initiated pending surgery, for an estimated median of 3 days. The duration of antibiotic treatment varies according to the initial presentation of the symptoms, which may begin with an isolated fever for which there is no explanation, or a local condition in which there is some doubt as to the depth of involvement. Although antibiotic therapy is a cornerstone of treatment, it must always be combined with surgical debridement as soon as possible(14,17) in order to limit the spread of the infectious process.

1.4.5. Radiological findings

The use of imaging to diagnose mediastinitis is still a subject of debate.

Because of low specificity and low sensitivity, differentiation between a postoperative status judged to be 'normal' and the presence of stigmata of infection is very difficult, especially in the early postoperative period (14-21 days on average)(7,8,12,42). Infiltration of the mediastinal fat, the presence of retrosternal collections which may correspond to a hematoma or sedeme, pericardial or pleural effusion are described but with low specificity(7,8,12,42).

Foldyna et al(42) compared the postoperative CT data of patients who developed mediastinitis with those who had simple sequelae in 105 patients, and showed that the presence of free gas bubbles, pleural effusions and the size of the brachiocephalic lymph nodes were independently associated with infectious mediastinitis.

The presence of air bubbles appears to be the most specific sign in the literature(7,8), followed by sternal separation.

There is also evidence that CT is more cost-effective in cases of late infection or recurrence(7,8,12).

It should be noted that all these scan data must be correlated with the clinical-biological pictures and under no circumstances should they delay the resumption of surgery.

1.4.6. Biological elements

We analysed the white blood cell count, CRP and procalcitonin as markers of infection and the pre-operative haemoglobin level.

The lowest median post-CEC hemoglobin level was 8.9g/dl with a minimum of 6.9g/dl. Post-ECC anaemia and recourse to transfusion, widely described in the literature, constitute risk factors for the genesis of infection by altering the healing process. Some authors recommend a hemoglobin level of at least 10g/dl to ensure satisfactory healing(53-56).

Siciliano et al(7) established in their study that a white blood cell count above 14,000 (equivalent to that found in our series) multiplies the risk by 2.5, whereas this limit was lower for Foldyna et al(42) and Kallel et al(12) (10,000).

The median CRP in our series was 213, higher than that reported by Foldyna et al(42).

It should be noted that these values are analysed according to the clinical context, and it is rather the kinetics that are of diagnostic value(17,51). In the case of some patients with an early-onset infection, it is sometimes difficult to distinguish between post-CEC SIRS and infection(57,58).

As a result, the diagnostic importance of procalcitonin in differentiating between a bacterial infectious process and an inflammatory process(8,12,57,58).

2. Intraoperative data

2.1. Different stages of the operation

The cornerstone of treatment is effective antibiotic therapy followed by early surgical debridement(4).

Surgical treatment has clear imperatives:

- Treating sepsis
- Debriding
- Stabilising the sternum
- Closure of the wound(59,60)

2.2. Installation

The patient is positioned supine, with a cross-bar under the shoulder blades to facilitate exposure. The upper limbs are aligned alongside the body. The operating field always includes the two femoral trigones up to mid-thigh. Under general anaesthetic.

2.2.1. Operating procedure

Controlling the source of infection and debridement of infected tissue are the cornerstones of surgical treatment for mediastinitis.

Although the most appropriate surgical approach for the treatment of mediastinitis is still under debate, there is consensus that at the very least the wound should be debrided.

Surgery consists of mediastinal exploration through the old sternotomy incision.

A curettage of the fibrin deposits is carried out together with a trimming of the skin and subcutaneous tissues.

Multiple bacteriological samples were taken. Non-vascularised areas of the sternum were resected. Finally, the pericardial cavity was cleaned and the mediastinal region was abundantly irrigated with Betadine serum diluted to 0.5%.

A drainage system is put in place and finally the sternum is synthesised.

2.3. Sternal closure techniques

Two approaches are the most common for closing the wound:

(i) Primary intention, i.e. the wound is closed by bringing the edges together

(ii) Tertiary intention or delayed primary closure, i.e. the wound is debrided and left open for treatment and observation, then closed a few days later.

(iii) However, a secondary intention approach, i.e. there is no direct closure and the wound granulates and heals, is rarely used(59-62).

None of the patients in our series had delayed closure; they all had closure in the same operative time, given that sternal stability was still ensured and the loss of substances was manageable.

Sternal instability leads to local tissue necrosis with increased movement of the bone table, which in turn triggers bacterial growth. Conversely, stable sternal fixation reduces the frequency of tissue trauma and promotes revascularisation and bone consolidation.

In fact, a correct median sternotomy reduces the occurrence of sternal instability and dehiscence, whereas a paramedian sternotomy, whatever the sternal closure technique, can be a source of sternal instability.

In our population, the initial closure after bypass surgery was almost always a conventional closure using single-circle para-sternal steel wires.

After recovery, the technique differs depending on the local condition and the associated risk factors.

In fact, 54% of cases had a simple closure associated in 33% of cases with a "figure of eight" or "X" closure, and 47% had a closure using the modified Robicsek technique (the para-sternal frame).

Numerous studies compare closure techniques with regard to sternal biomechanics(63-66), efficacy in high-risk patients(63,67) and the rate of complications(68), in particular sternal dehiscence or mediastinitis.

And surprisingly, there y been a lack of research into postoperative patient comfort, pain and readaptation rates compared to the surgical closure technique after median sternotomy.

Whichever method is chosen, the steel wires used to close the sternum can be passed around the sternum, through the intercostal spaces (para sternal, the method chosen in our department) or through the sternum (trans sternal).

Sternal instability results from the sutures rubbing against the sternum due to the pressure exerted by its lateral edges. These pressures are theoretically much greater when the sutures are passed trans-sternal, although the results of series comparing the two techniques in the literature are controversial(1,2,32).

The current standard for the closure of sternotomies remains single-circle sutures, with two at the level of the sternal manubrium and the remainder for the sternal body(32,34).

Losanoff et al(64) compared the biomechanical properties of six sternal closures on 53 human cadaver models. They concluded that the mechanical stability of a single-strand closure was significantly superior to that of figure-of-eight closures.

Similarly, Schimmer et al(68) carried out a prospective randomised clinical trial on a group of 339 patients, which included a subgroup of elderly patients (over 75 years of age) with a higher risk of wound healing complications. The trial showed no statistically significant difference between the closure techniques evaluated (conventional and Robicsek).

Figure-of-eight closure techniques appear to increase the strength and stability of sternal closures by minimising longitudinal movements, and in osteoporotic patients (avoid cutting wires in contact with the sternal margin) (1,34,69).

In a randomised trial published by Bottio et al(70) involving 700 high-risk patients and comparing single versus figure-of-eight closure, figure-of-eight closure was associated with a significantly reduced incidence of deep and superficial infections.

In an Asian observational study published by Abdul-Rahman et al(71) comparing 7835 patients in whom figure-of-eight wires were used with 2122 patients in whom the conventional technique was used, the incidence of dehiscence was significantly lower in the figure-of-eight group.

Although the results of figure-of-eight closures remain uncertain for some patients, there is evidence that the modified Robicsek technique for patients with multiple fractures and those with increased risk factors represents a good alternative by reducing the incidence of sternal dehiscence and infections(9,34,59,68).

The technique described by Robicsek and colleagues in 1977 has several advantages: it stabilises the sternum in the event of fragility or breakage, even if subsequent instability develops, and it prevents the wires from shearing the bone. In fact, it transfers the pressure site by changing the contact point from metal to bone to metal to metal, thereby providing broader support(9,67,68).

The disadvantage of this technique is that it produces a constrictive weave which can disrupt the collateral blood supply to the sternum, and effective consolidation of the upper and lower sternum beant cannot be achieved. Indeed, the original technique was modified by Sutherland and colleagues and Sharma and colleagues(2,63,68,72), who placed a continuous steel wire on each side of the sternum and tied the two lines cranially and caudally. This modification has an additional advantage over the conventional Robicsek closure, in that the blood supply to the sternum is not "angled".

In a study by Molina and colleagues(73), 123 obese patients were prospectively divided into two groups (Robicsek technique, n 54, versus standard sternal closure, n 69). The group using the Robicsek technique had no dehiscence (0%), compared with 6 dehiscences (8.7%) in the group using the standard closure.

Similarly, Sharma and colleagues (74) showed in 776 high-risk patients (390 conventional closure versus 386 closure with the modified Robicsek technique) that the incidence of postoperative sternal wound complications was significantly higher, 16 patients, for those closed using the conventional technique versus one patient in patients treated with the new technique.

Rigid sternal fixation techniques include a wide range of bands, hooks and sternal plates. Results are mixed. Some studies have shown that rigid fixation reduces pain while providing better sternal stability in high-risk patients, but others have reported that rigid sternal fixation does not alter the risk of scarring or infection(l,59,62,68,72,75-78).

It should be noted that these techniques are more expensive. Elies are contraindicated in patients with osteoporosis or active infection. Elies are not indicated for uncomplicated sternal closures and should only be used in high-risk patients(l,59,62,68,72,75-78).

The median number of steel wires used in our series was 6 wires. Some authors have shown that there was an inverse relationship between the number of wire bands and the infection rate(l,32,59,79).

Another closure technique widely described in the literature, and recently introduced, is VACtherapy (Vacuum Assisted Closure).

First described by Davydov in 1992 and applied in surgery by Argenta and Morykwas in 1997, it was initially used to treat bedsores and chronic ulcers. Since then, its use has been extended to other types of chronic wound, particularly post-operative.

The first studies describing its use in cardiac surgery date back to 2000(80,81).

It is used alone or in conjunction with surgical treatment or hydrocellular dressings.

After surgical debridement, the system is fitted. It consists of a sponge, usually made of polyurethane with a pore size ranging from 400 to 600pm, mounted on a drainage system connected to a source of negative pressure capable of generating pressures of 25 to 200mmhg. Watertightness is ensured by an adhesive system covering the wound and extending 4-6 cm beyond it(80-85).

The dressing is changed every 48 hours under rigorous aseptic conditions, with the wound checked and bacteriological samples taken. Suction may be discontinued as soon as the amount of exudate has decreased, and the dressing may be changed after more than 48 hours (83).

2.4. Post-surgical drainage

Closure on a drainage system consisting of two or three drains.

This will be used to aspirate the often abundant exudates, and to inject a saline solution on a daily basis, combined with an antiseptic with or without antibiotics.

Post-operative drainage, whether by rendon drains or №32 drains with an associated suction system, is usually combined with the two systems together and y kept to a maximum, in fact the median duration was estimated at lOjours for all patients.

3. Post-operative data
3.1. Stay

58% of our patients required a stay in intensive care after revision surgery, 26% of whom had already been diagnosed in intensive care.

Being an inflammatory and septic process, septic shock developed in 45% of patients, necessitating the use of catecholamines.

We have not found any studies detailing the after-effects of the operation in terms of resuscitation.

The estimated length of stay in intensive care after surgery is 3 days, with an average of 8 days and a range from one day to two months.

The prolonged stay was mainly due to septic shock. Other complications were noted, such as pulmonary infection, altered neurological status, respiratory distress requiring intubation, or already prolonged intubation.

The total length of stay for patients with mediastinitis was obviously longer, estimated at 42 days.

This prolonged hospitalisation, the specific resuscitation is costly, the antibiotic treatment is long, the care is multiplied and there are many people involved, all of which has a heavy impact on the health economy.

3.2. Bacteriological data

In 55.6% of patients, a germ was identified, mainly from the Staphylococcus family: staphylococcus aureus or coagulase-negative staphylococcus.

As with any infection, mediastinitis can be caused by multiple germs. The micro-organisms isolated from deep sternal infections are often staphylococci, S. aureus (40-60%) or coagulase-negative staphylococci (15-25%)(2,15,28,52). The percentage of methicillin-resistant strains depends on local prevalence. However, for coagulase-negative staphylococci, the proportion of resistant strains is over 70%(52,86,87). Gram-negative bacilli (GNB) are encountered more frequently in 20 to over 30% of cases in certain studies(52). Among these BGN infections, it is not uncommon to find multi-resistant strains such as those carrying a broad-spectrum betalactamase (ESBL).

Similarly, the presence of enterococci, mainly Enterococcus faecalis, is regularly reported in the literature, representing up to 10% of the causative agents(52).

B. Gardlund et al, in their study of 126 cases of mediastinitis, proposed the nature of the germ according to the clinical data.

In fact, three fundamentally different types have been distinguished: (1) mediastinitis associated with obesity and sternal dehiscence, sometimes also with chronic obstructive pulmonary disease, and often caused by coagulase-negative staphylococci, (2) mediastinitis following intraoperative contamination of the mediastinal space often caused by S. aureus, and (3) mediastinitis due to the spread of concomitant infections to sites other than the mediastinum during the postoperative period, often caused by gram-negative bacilli(52).

Local changes in the distribution of the main germs should be taken into account when initiating probabilistic antibiotic treatment.

Other micro-organisms may be involved very rarely (< 1%): this is the case with yeasts (Candida), often in particularly immunocompromised patients (transplants) or in mediastinitis initially caused by bacteria and treated with antibiotics. The other germs are "curiosities", the source of numerous clinical cases in the medical literature, but whose actual incidence is negligible(88,89).

3.3. Local complications

The evolution of the surgical wound is one of the main criteria used to assess the success of the surgery in the first instance and the management protocol in general.

Unfortunately, in some cases it becomes chronic. The factors precipitating this unfavourable evolution are numerous and still poorly elucidated.

Due to a failure to sterilise the site of infection during the surgical procedure, or secondary contamination from the patient's flora (colonised by multi-resistant hospital germs after a prolonged stay), or from the environment (especially handling).

In our series, persistent infection affected 12 patients, i.e. 26% of the population.

In the form of fistulisation of the skin, discharge or loss of skin substance.

either involvement of the supra-sternal planes (superficial involvement) or recurrence of a deep infection.

Recurrence of mediastinitis is a very rare occurrence, and four patients in our series required repeat surgery.

This is a major turning point in the clinical course. The disease is often more severe, with multi-resistant germs, and treatment is often very delabrant. The results are disappointing and the mortality rate is very high.

There are several drawbacks to this system:

A third operation for the patient, often very difficult to accept.

The difficulty of closure at a multi-operation site, with fragile, inflexible tissues and often significant parietal tension. And considering the seriousness of the surgical revision itself, given the posterior adhesions between the sternum and the mediastinal structures, particularly after coronary bypass surgery, where sternotomy is associated in 1040% of cases with graft lesions, fatal in 50% of cases(80). There have even been reports of rupture of the right ventricle, which is anatomically thin and weakened by the infectious episode(80).

The drainage system is cumbersome for the patient, the first lift is delayed and ambulation is often difficult for the patient. These complications will further complicate the post-operative period and cause great physical and moral harm to the patient.

II. Analytical study of postoperative mortality due to mediastinitis

The univariate study identified several risk factors described as being predictive of mortality:

age over 70, and obesity.

Post-ECC cardiac dysfunction, altered neurological status, the development of sepsis or septic shock requiring the use of catecholamines, hemodialysis and the need for reintubation.

Diagnosis during the stay in intensive care, and a prolonged stay in intensive care beyond 48 hours post-CEC.

Recurrence of infection and the need for a third operation. The development of sepsis or septic shock at the time of diagnosis.

In recent years, there have not been many studies looking at risk factors for mediastinal mortality, although a few have been identified in the literature.

The majority of studies have focused on risk factors for mediastinitis.

However, a few have been identified in the literature.

Table XXX Hospital mortality reported in the various studies

Author	Reference	Annëe	Number of inhabitants	Death rate^
Wu et al	(14)	2016	2,835	12%
Trouillet et al	(90)	2005	316	20.3%
Lepelletier et al	(91)	2009	39	12.8%
Karra et al	(92)	2006	183	27%
Gatti et al	(25)	2018	142	5.6%
Dubert et al	(51)	2015	160	20%

Trouillet et al(90) proved through their study by applying a logistic regression analysis, five factors independently associated with mortality in the intensive care unit:

Age over 70, the nature of the initial operation, mechanical ventilation for more than 72 hours, and persistent positive bacteremia.

With the exception of the nature of the CEC, the other factors were related to the severity of the underlying disease and the severity of the acute illnessë.

These factors multiply the risk of death by 3.

Another series by Karra et al (92), involving 183 patients, identified the factors predicting mortality at one year.

the factors identified were: delayed sternal closure (more than 72 hours) after revision surgery (risk multiplied by 6), age over 65 years (risk multiplied by 2), a serum creatinine level greater than 176 pmol/l before debridement (risk multiplied by 2),a stay in an intensive care unit prior to sternal debridement (risk multiplied by 6), and bacteremia due to methicillin-resistant Staphylococcus aureus (risk multiplied by 2).

Treatment with antibiotics with in vitro activity against the infectious pathogen within 7 days of initial debridement has been associated with a reduced risk of mortality(92).

As for Lepelletier et al(91), in their series of 39 patients treated for mediastinitis, the only factor identified as predictive of mortality was the presence of an associated co-infection.

The instantaneous risk of death was increased seven-fold in patients with an associated infection, notably pneumonia. These results were similar to those found in the study by Trouillet et al(90) where positive bacteremia was identified as a risk factor for mortality.

Comparing these data with those found in our study, we identified four independent factors predictive of mortality:

age over 60, a post-CEC ventilation time of over 4 hours, admission in a critical state defined as cardiogenic or septic shock, the need for catecholamines, and finally (alteration of cardiac function at diagnosis).

These results appear to be consistent with those found in the literature. The advanced age, although the threshold changes according to the epidemiological nature of the population studied, reflects the fragility of the terrain through the associated comorbidities which will be an aggravating factor added to the complexity of the operative procedure and the post-operative sequelae.

The critical state, cardiac dysfunction and prolonged ventilation reflect the severity of the initial pathology, whether or not associated with the severity of the additional infection.

Delayed closure was not identified in our series as all patients had closure at the same operative time.

5 CONCLUSION

Mediastinitis is a serious post-sternotomy infectious complication, which increases the length of hospital stay, leads to higher costs and causes a significant increase in mortality.

The present work is a retrospective and descriptive study carried out in the cardio-thoracic surgery department of the HMPIT which collected data during the period from January 2010 to December 2019, including 55 patients.

The aims of this work were to :

- Describe the characteristics of patients who have developed this complication.
- Identify the risk factors for mortality.

The results of our study show that the mortality rate among patients who developed mediastinitis was 31%.

There are factors that contribute to morbidity and mortality, some of which are linked to the patient's condition and the circumstances and conditions of the operation.

Those linked to the patient, age over 60.

Good left ventricular function as a protective factor.

Those linked to the initial operation, concerning the post-operative after-effects, with a duration of ventilation in excess of 4 hours also seen as a protective factor.

And finally, admission in a critical condition as a risk factor.

In our series, the causative organisms were mainly staphylococci. For some patients, the infection itself and the development of a state of septic shock were not the direct causes of death, but rather favouring factors in a fragile environment.

Prolonged stays in intensive care, and the sometimes excessive use of antibiotics, can delay diagnosis and result in poor management.

The time it takes to get treatment is an important prognostic factor in limiting the damage and the spread of infection.

A better understanding of these factors would enable appropriate measures to be taken to reduce the incidence of this infection.

Preventive measures must therefore be put in place in every cardiac surgery department:

Raising the awareness of operating theatre staff, strict compliance with basic hygiene rules, the introduction of antibiotic prophylaxis adapted to the ecosystem, early diagnosis and timely surgical debridement are in themselves essential prognostic factors.

6 BIBLIOGRAPHIES

1. Jayakumar S, Khoynezhad A, Jahangiri M. Surgical Site Infections in Cardiac Surgery. Critical Care Clinics, Oct 2020;36(4):581-92.

2. Pradeep A, Rangasamy J, Varma PK. Recent developments in controlling sternal wound infection after cardiac surgery and measures to enhance sternal healing. Med Res Rev. March 2021;41(2):709-24.

3. Lemaignen A, Birgand G, Ghodhbane W, Alkhoder S, Lolom I, Belorgey S, et al. Sternal wound infection after cardiac surgery: incidence and risk factors according to clinical presentation. Clinical Microbiology and Infection, Jul 2015;21(7):674.ell-674.el8.

4. Pastene B, Cassir N, Tankel J, Einav S, Fournier PE, Thomas P, et al. Mediastinitis in the intensive care unit patient: a narrative review. Clinical Microbiology and Infection, Jan 2020;26(l):26-34.

5. van Wingerden JJ, de Mol BA, van der Horst CM. Defining post-sternotomy mediastinitis for clinical evidence-based studies. Asian Cardiovasc Thorac Ann. May 2016;24(4):355-63.

6. Mehaffey JH, Hawkins RB, Byler M, Charles EJ, Fonner C, Kron I, et al. Cost of individual complications following coronary artery bypass grafting. The Journal of Thoracic and Cardiovascular Surgery, March 2018;155(3):875- 882.el.

7. Siciliano RF, Medina ACR, Bittencourt MS, Gualandro D, Uezumi KK, Santos MVB, et al. Derivation and validation of an early diagnostic score for mediastinitis after cardiothoracic surgery. International Journal of Infectious Diseases, Jan 2020;90:201-5.

8. van Wingerden JJ, Maas M, Braam RL, de Mol BA. Diagnosing poststernotomy mediastinitis in the ED. The American Journal of Emergency Medicine, March 2016;34(3):618-22.

9. Fu RH, Weinstein AL, Chang MM, Argenziano M, Ascherman JA, Rohde CH. Risk factors of infected sternal wounds versus sterile wound dehiscence. Journal of Surgical Research.Jan2016;200(l):400-7.

10. Reser D, Caliskan E, Tolboom H, Guidotti A, Maisano F. Median sternotomy. MMCTS. 2015;2015:mmv017.

11. Ma JG, An JX. Deep sternal wound infection after cardiac surgery: a comparison of three different wound infection types and an analysis of antibiotic resistance. J Thorac Dis. Jan 2018;10(l):377-87.

12. Kallel S, Abdenadher M, Ellouze M, Cheikhrouhou H, Triki Z, Maaloul I, et al. Mediastinitis after cardiac surgery: incidence, risk factors, prognosis and prevention. 2013;10.

13. Oliveira F dos S, Freitas LDO de, Rabelo-Silva ER, Costa LM da, Kalil RAK,

Moraes MAP de. Predictors of Mediastinitis Risk after Coronary Artery Bypass Surgery: Applicability of Score in 1,322 Cases. Arquivos Brasileiros de Cardiologia ,Arq Bras Cardiol. 2017; 109(3):207-212.

14. Wu L, Chung KC, Waljee JF, Momoh AO, Zhong L, Sears ED. A National Study of the Impact of Initial Debridement Timing on Outcomes for Patients with Deep Sternal Wound Infection: Plastic and Reconstructive Surgery, Feb 2016;137(2):414e-23e.

15. Nieminen VJ, Jaaskelainen IH, Eklund AM, Murto ES, Mattila KJ, Juvonen TS, et al. The characteristics of postoperative mediastinitis duringthe changing phases of cardiac surgery. The Annals of Thoracic Surgery. j.athoracsur.2020.10.029.

16. O'Brien SM, Feng L, He X, Xian Y, Jacobs JP, Badhwar V, et al. The Society of Thoracic Surgeons 2018 Adult Cardiac Surgery Risk Models: Part 2- Statistical Methods and Results. The Annals of Thoracic Surgery, May 2018;105(5):1419-28.

17. Chan M, Yusuf E, Giulieri S, Perrottet N, Von Segesser L, Borens 0, et al. A retrospective study of deep sternal wound infections: clinical and microbiological characteristics, treatment, and risk factors for complications. Diagnostic Microbiology and Infectious Disease, March 2016;84(3):261-5.

18. Nieto-Cabrera M, Fernandez-Perez C, Garcia-Gonzalez I, Martin-Benitez JC, Ferrero J, Bringas M, et al. Med-Score 24: A multivariable prediction model for poststernotomy mediastinitis 24 hours after admission to the intensive care unit. The Journal of Thoracic and Cardiovascular Surgery, March 2018;155(3):1041-1051.e5.

19. Conti V. Poststernotomy mediastinitis: Early risk factors identified but hard to modify. The Journal of Thoracic and Cardiovascular Surgery, March 2018;155(3):1052.

20. Ouerchefani A. Mediastinitis after cardiac surgery: A propos de 18 cases. La tunisie chirurgicale - 2015 ; Vol 25.

21. Wang B, He D, Wang M, Qian Y, Lu Y, Shi X, et al. Analysis of sternal healing after median sternotomy in low-risk patients at midterm follow-up: retrospective cohort study from two centres. J Cardiothorac Surg. Dec 2019;14(l):193.

22. Ghannem M, Ahmaidi S, Ghannem L, Meimoun P. Infectious and inflammatory complications after cardiac surgery in cardiac rehabilitation units. Annales de Cardiologie et d'Angeiologie. Dec 2020;69(6):424-9.

23. Raja SG, Rochon M, Jarman JWE. Brompton Harefield Infection Score (BHIS): development and validation of a stratification tool for predicting risk of surgical site infection after coronary artery bypass grafting. International Journal of Surgery, Apr 2015;16:69-73.

24. Biancari F, Gatti G, Rosato S, Mariscalco G, Pappalardo A, Onorati F, et al.

Preoperative risk stratification of deep sternal wound infection after coronary surgery. Infect Control Hosp Epidemiol, Apr 2020;41(4):444-51.

25. Gatti G, Benussi B, Brunetti D, Ceschia A, Porcari A, Biondi F, et al. The fate of patients having deep sternal infection after bilateral internal thoracic artery grafting in the negative pressure wound therapy era. International Journal of Cardiology, Oct 2018;269:67-74.

26. Phoon PHY, Hwang NC. Deep Sternal Wound Infection: Diagnosis, Treatment and Prevention. Journal of Cardiothoracic and Vascular Anesthesia, June 2020;34(6):1602-13.

27. Gatti G, Maschietto L, Morosin M, Russo M, Benussi B, Forti G, et al. Routine use of bilateral internal thoracic artery grafting in women: A risk factor analysis for poor outcomes. Cardiovascular Revascularization Medicine, Jan 2017;18(l):40-6.

28. Risnes I, Abdelnoor M, Almdahl SM, Svennevig JL. Mediastinitis After Coronary Artery Bypass Grafting Risk Factors and Long-Term Survival. The Annals ofThoracic Surgery, May 2010;89(5):1502-9.

29. Gummert JF, Barten MJ, Hans C, Kluge M, Doll N, Walther T, et al. Mediastinitis and Cardiac Surgery - an Updated Risk Factor Analysis in 10,373 Consecutive Adult Patients. Thorac cardiovasc Surg. Apr 2002;50(2):87-91.

30. Filsoufi F, Castillo JG, Rahmanian PB, Broumand SR, Silvay G, Carpentier A, et al. Epidemiology of Deep Sternal Wound Infection in Cardiac Surgery. Journal of Cardiothoracic and Vascular Anesthesia, August 2009;23(4):488-94.

31. Rehman SM, Elzain O, Mitchell J, Shine B, Bowler ICJW, Sayeed R, et al. Risk factors for mediastinitis following cardiac surgery: the importance of managing obesity. Journal of Hospital Infection, Oct 2014;88(2):96-102.

32. Shaikhrezai K, Robertson FL, Anderson SE, Slight RD, Brackenbury ET. Does the number of wires used to close a sternotomy have an impact on deep sternal wound infection? Interactive Cardiovascular and Thoracic Surgery. 1 Aug 2012;15(2):219-22.

33. Cayci C, Russo M, Cheema F, Martens T, Ozcan V, Argenziano M, et al. Risk Analysis of Deep Sternal Wound Infections and Their Impact on Long-Term Survival: A Propensity Analysis. Annals of Plastic Surgery, Sept 2008;61(3):294-301.

34. Lazar HL, Salm TV, Engelman R, Orgill D, Gordon S. Prevention and management of sternal wound infections. The Journal of Thoracic and Cardiovascular Surgery, Oct 2016;152(4):962-72.

35. Yumun G, Erdolu B, Toktas F, Eris C, Ay D, Turk T, et al. Deep Sternal Wound Infection after Coronary Artery Bypass Surgery: Management and Risk Factor Analysis for Mortality. HSF. Sep 1, 2014;17(4):212.

36. Ali U, Bibo L, Pierre M, Bayfield N, Raichel L, Merry C, et al. Deep Sternal

Wound Infections After Cardiac Surgery: A New Australian Tertiary Centre Experience. Heart, Lung and Circulation, Oct 2020;29(10):1571-8.

37. Perrault LP, Kirkwood KA, Chang HL, Mullen JC, Gulack BC, Argenziano M, et al. A Prospective Multi-Institutional Cohort Study of Mediastinal Infections After Cardiac Operations. The Annals of Thoracic Surgery, Feb 2018;105(2):461-8.

38. Fakih MG, Sharma M, Khatib R, Berriel-Cass D, Meisner S, Harrington S, et al. Increase in the Rate of Sternal Surgical Site Infection After Coronary Artery Bypass Graft: A Marker of Higher Severity of Illness. Infect Control Hosp Epidemiol, June 2007;28(6):655-60.

39. Dai C, Lu Z, Zhu H, Xue S, Lian F. Bilateral Internal Mammary Artery Grafting and Risk of Sternal Wound Infection: Evidence From Observational Studies. The Annals of Thoracic Surgery, June 2013;95(6):1938-45.

40. Raza S, Blackstone EH, Houghtaling PL, Koprivanac M, Ravichandren K, Javadikasgari H, et al. Similar Outcomes in Diabetes Patients After Coronary Artery Bypass Grafting With Single Internal Thoracic Artery Plus Radial Artery Grafting and Bilateral Internal Thoracic Artery Grafting. The Annals of Thoracic Surgery, Dec 2017;104(6):1923-32.

41. Leung Wai Sang S, Chaturvedi R, Alam A, Samoukovic G, deVarennes B, Lachapelle K. Preoperative hospital length of stay as a modifiable risk factor for mediastinitis after cardiac surgery. J Cardiothorac Surg. dec 2013;8(I):45.

42. Foldyna B, Mueller M, Etz CD, Luecke C, Haunschild J, Hoffmann I, et al. Computed tomography improves the differentiation of infectious mediastinitis from normal postoperative changes after sternotomy in cardiac surgery. Eur Radiol, June 2019;29(6):2949-57.

43. Abdelnoor M, Sandven I, Vengen O, Risnes I. Mediastinitis in open heart surgery: a systematic review and meta-analysis of risk factors. Scandinavian CardiovascularJournal. 3 Sep 2019;53(5):226-34.

44. Vrancic JM, Piccinini F, Camporrotondo M, Espinoza JC, Camou JI, Nacinovich F, et al. Bilateral Internal Thoracic Artery Grafting Increases Mediastinitis: Myth or Fact? The Annals ofThoracic Surgery, March 2017;103(3):834-9.

45. Deo SV, Shah IK, Dunlay SM, Erwin PJ, Locker C, Altarabsheh SE, et al. Bilateral Internal Thoracic Artery Harvest and Deep Sternal Wound Infection in Diabetic Patients. The Annals ofThoracic Surgery, March 2013;95(3):862-9.

46. Ruka E, Dagenais F, Mohammadi S, Chauvette V, Poirier P, Voisine P. Bilateral mammary artery grafting increases postoperative mediastinitis without survival benefit in obese patients. Eur J Cardiothorac Surg. dec 2016;50(6):1188-95.

47. Hirahara N, Miyata H, Motomura N, Kohsaka S, Nishimura T, Takamoto S. Procedure- and Hospital-Level Variation of Deep Sternal Wound Infection From

All-Japan Registry. The Annals of Thoracic Surgery, Feb 2020;109(2):547-54.

48. Lu J. Risk factors for sternal wound infection and mid-term survival following coronary artery bypass surgery. European Journal of Cardio-Thoracic Surgery.June 2003;23(6):943-9.

49. Oliveira F dos S, Freitas LDO de, Rabelo-Silva ER, Costa LM da, Kalil RAK, Moraes MAP de. Predictors of Mediastinitis Risk after Coronary Artery Bypass Surgery: Applicability of Score in 1,322 Cases. Arquivos Brasileiros de Cardiologia Arq Bras Cardiol. 2017; 109(3):207-212.

50. Juan R, Aguado JM, Lopez MJ, Lumbreras C, Enriquez F, Sanz F, et al. Accuracy of blood culture for early diagnosis of mediastinitis in febrile patients after cardiac surgery. Eur J Clin Microbiol Infect Dis. March 2005;24(3):182-9.

51. Dubert M, Pourbaix A, Alkhoder S, Mabileau G, Lescure FX, Ghodhbane W, et al. Sternal Wound Infection after Cardiac Surgery: Management and Outcome. Yang F, editor. PLoS ONE. 30 Sep 2015;10(9):e0139122.

52. Ga B. Postoperative mediastinitis in cardiac surgery - microbiology and pathogenesisq. Thoracic Surgery. 2002;6.

53. Ang LB, Veloria EN, Evanina EY, Smaldone A. Mediastinitis and blood transfusion in cardiac surgery: A systematic review. Heart & Lung, May 2012;41(3):255-63.

54. Abukhodair AW, Alqarni MS, Bukhari ZM, Qadi A, Mufti HN, Fernandez JA, et al. Association Between Post-Operative Infection and Blood Transfusion in Cardiac Surgery. Cureus Jul 2020; 12(7): e8985.

55. Horvath KA, Acker MA, Chang H, Bagiella E, Smith PK, Iribarne A, et al. Blood Transfusion and Infection After Cardiac Surgery. The Annals of Thoracic Surgery, June 2013;95(6):2194-201.

56. Patel NN, Avlonitis VS, Jones HE, Reeves BC, Sterne JAC, Murphy GJ. Indications for red blood cell transfusion in cardiac surgery: a systematic review and meta-analysis. The Lancet Haematology. dec 2015;2(12):e543-53.

57. Evora PRB, Bottura C, Arcencio L, Albuquerque AAS, Evora PM, Rodrigues AJ. Key Points for Curbing Cardiopulmonary Bypass Inflammation. Acta Cir Bras. 2016;31(suppl I):45-52.

58. Aljure OD, Fabbro M. Cardiopulmonary Bypass and Inflammation: The Hidden Enemy. Journal of Cardiothoracic and Vascular Anesthesia, Feb 2019;33(2):346-7.

59. Lonie S, Hallam J, Yii M, Davis P, Newcomb A, Nixon I, et al. Changes in the management of deep sternal wound infections: a 12-year review: Deep sternal wound infection management. ANZ J Surg. Nov 2015;85(II):878-81.

60. Goh SSC. Post-sternotomy mediastinitis in the modern era. J Card Surg. Sep 2017;32(9):556-66.

61. Fleck TM, Koller R, Giovanoli P, Moidl R, Czerny M, Fleck M, et al. Primary or Delayed Closure for the Treatment of Poststernotomy Wound Infections: Annals of Plastic Surgery, March 2004;52(3):310-4.

62. Levin LS, Miller AS, Gajjar AH, Bremer KD, Spann J, Milano CA, et al. An Innovative Approach for Sternal Closure. The Annals of Thoracic Surgery, June 2010;89(6):1995-9.

63. Kukulski L, Krawczyk A, Pacholewicz J. Retrospective analysis of the impact of sternum closure technique on postoperative comfort and rehabilitation, kitp. 2018;15(4):233-7.

64. Losanoff JE, Collier AD, Wagner-Mann CC, Richman BW, Huff H, Hsieh F hung, et al. Biomechanical comparison of median sternotomy closures. The Annals of Thoracic Surgery, Jan 2004;77(l):203-9.

65. McGregor WE, Trumble DR, Magovern JA. Mechanical analysis of midline sternotomy wound closure. The Journal of Thoracic and Cardiovascular Surgery, June 1999;117(6):1144-50.

66. Casha AR, Gauci M, Yang L, Saleh M, Kay PH, Cooper GJ. Fatigue testing median sternotomy closuresq. Thoracic Surgery. 2001;5.

67. Schimmer C, Sommer SP, Bensch M, Bohrer T, Aleksic I, Leyh R. Sternal closure techniques and postoperative sternal wound complications in elderly patients. European Journal of Cardio-Thoracic Surgery, July 2008;34(l):132-8.

68. Schimmer C, Reents W, Berneder S, Eigel P, Sezer O, Scheid H, et al. Prevention of Sternal Dehiscence and Infection in High-Risk Patients: A Prospective Randomized Multicenter Trial. The Annals of Thoracic Surgery, Dec 2008;86(6):1897-904.

69. Pradeep et al - 2021 - Recent developments in controlling sternal wound. Med Res Rev. March 2021;41(2):709-24.

70. Bottio T, Rizzoli G, Vida V, Casarotto D, Gerosa G. Double crisscross sternal wiring and chest wound infections: A prospective randomized study. The Journal of Thoracic and Cardiovascular Surgery, Nov 2003;126(5):1352-6.

71. Ramzisham ARM, Raflis AR, Khairulasri MG, Min JOS, Fikri AM, Zamrin MD. Figure-of-Eight vs. Interrupted Sternal Wire Closure of Median Sternotomy. Asian Cardiovasc Thorac Ann. Dec 2009;17(6):587-91.

72. Kaul P. Sternal reconstruction after post-sternotomy mediastinitis. J Cardiothorac Surg. dec 2017;12(l):94.

73. Molina JE, Lew RSL, Hyland KJ. Postoperative sternal dehiscence in obese patients: Incidence and prevention. The Annals of Thoracic Surgery, Sept 2004;78(3):912-7.

74. Sharma R, Puri D, Panigrahi BP, Virdi IS. A modified parasternal wire technique

for prevention and treatment of sternal dehiscence. The Annals ofThoracic Surgery, Jan 2004;77(I):210-3.

75. Fawzy H, Osei-Tutu K, Errett L, Latter D, Bonneau D, Musgrave M, et al. Sternal plate fixation for sternal wound reconstruction: initial experience (Retrospective study). J Cardiothorac Surg. Dec 2011;6(I):63.

76. Cicilioni OJ, Stieg FH, Papanicolaou G. Sternal Wound Reconstruction with Transverse Plate Fixation: Plastic and Reconstructive Surgery, Apr 2005;115(5):1297-303.

77. Wang B, He D, Wang M, Qian Y, Lu Y, Shi X, et al. Analysis ofsternal healing after median sternotomy in low-risk patients at midterm follow-up: retrospective cohort study from two centres. J Cardiothorac Surg. Dec 2019;14(I):193.

78. Liao JM, Chan P, Cornwell L, Tsai PI, Joo JH, Bakaeen FG, et al. Feasibility of primary sternal plating for morbidly obese patients after cardiac surgery. J Cardiothorac Surg. dec 2019;14(I):25.

79. Zeitani J, de Peppo AP, Moscarelli M, Wolf LG, Scafuri A, Nardi P, et al. Influence of sternal size and inadvertent paramedian sternotomy on stability of the closure site: A clinical and mechanical study. The Journal of Thoracic and Cardiovascular Surgery, July 2006;132(I):38-42.

80. Sartipy U, Lockowandt U, Gabel J, Jideus L, Dellgren G. Cardiac Rupture During Vacuum-Assisted Closure Therapy. The Annals of Thoracic Surgery, Sept 2006;82(3):1110-I.

81. Domkowski PW, Smith ML, Gonyon DL, Drye C, Wooten MK, Levin LS, et al. Evaluation of vacuum-assisted closure in the treatment of poststernotomy mediastinitis. The Journal of Thoracic and Cardiovascular Surgery, August 2003;126(2):386-9.

82. Bapat V, El-Muttardi N, Young C, Venn G, Roxburgh J. Experience with Vacuum-Assisted Closure of Sternal Wound Infections Following Cardiac Surgery and Evaluation of Chronic Complications Associated with its Use. J Cardiac Surgery, May 2008;23(3):227-33.

83. Falagas ME, Tansarli GS, Kapaskelis A, Vardakas KZ. Impact of Vacuum-Assisted Closure (VAC) Therapy on Clinical Outcomes of Patients with Sternal Wound Infections: A Meta-Analysis of Non-Randomized Studies. Landoni G, editor. PLoS ONE. 31 May 2013;8(5):e64741.

84. Mokhtari A, Sjogren J, Nilsson J, Gustafsson R, Malmsjo M, Ingemansson R. The cost of vacuum-assisted closure therapy in treatment of deep sternal wound infection. Scandinavian Cardiovascular Journal. Jan 2008;42(I):85-9.

85. Cowan KN, Teague L, Sue SC, Mahoney JL. Vacuum-Assisted Wound Closure of Deep Sternal Infections in High-Risk Patients After Cardiac Surgery. The Annals

ofThoracic Surgery, Dec 2005;80(6):2205-12.

86. Bennett-Guerrero E. Effect of an Implantable Gentamicin-Collagen Sponge on Sternal Wound Infections Following Cardiac SurgeryA Randomized Trial. JAMA. August 18, 2010;304(7):755.

87. Lytsy B, Lindblom RPF, Ransjb U, Leo-Swenne C. Hygienic interventions to decrease deep sternal wound infections following coronary artery bypass grafting. Journal of Hospital Infection, Dec 2015;91(4):326-31.

88. Duployez C, Loiez C, Hund R, Jegou B, Decoene C, Wallet F. A case of bacteremic mediastinitis due to Prevotella buccae after cardiac surgery. Anaerobe, fevr 2020;61:102097.

89. Fernandez AL, Adrio B, Martinez Cereijo JM, Martinez Monzonis MA, El- Diasty MM, Alvarez Escudero J. Clinical study of an outbreak of postoperative mediastinitis caused by Serratia marcescens in adult cardiac surgery. Interactive Cardiovascular and Thoracic Surgery. 1 Apr 2020;30(4):523-7.

90. Trouillet JL, Vuagnat A, Combes A, Bors V, Chastre J, Gandjbakhch I, et al. Acute poststernotomy mediastinitis managed with debridement and closed-drainage aspiration: Factors associated with death in the intensive care unit. The Journal of Thoracic and Cardiovascular Surgery, March 2005;129(3):518-24.

91. Lepelletier D, Poupelin L, Corvee S, Bourigault C, Bizouarn P, Blanloeil Y, et al. Risk factors for mortality in patients with mediastinitis after cardiac surgery. Archives of Cardiovascular Diseases, Feb 2009;102(2):119-25.

92. Karra R, McDermott L, Connelly S, Smith P, Sexton DJ, Kaye KS. Risk factors for 1-year mortality after postoperative mediastinitis. The Journal of Thoracic and Cardiovascular Surgery, Sept 2006;132(3):537-43.

Appendix 1: Framework used :

1.   Preoperative data :

1.1. Demographics:

Age, sex, CML, smoking.

1.2. Antecedents:

1.2.1. Non-cardiac :

Diabetes: age and HbAlc level, obstructive bronchopneumonia, renal insufficiency and use of haemodialysis, premedication with corticoids or immunosuppressive treatment, the notion of thoracic irradiation, the presence of arteriopathy other than cardiac.

1.2.2. Cardiac :

CEC redux, hypertension, dyslipidemia.

The severity of post bypass heart disease: the contractile function of the LV associated or not with right ventricular dysfunction (TAPSE, S').

1.3. The nature of the initial operation :

Myocardial revascularisation: the number of vessels revascularised and the mono- or bi-mammary sampling, valve replacement or repair, combined revascularisation and valve surgery, infective endocarditis, other types of operation.

The duration of bypass surgery and the duration of aortic clamping.

Initial post-CEC ventilation time.

Euroscore II.

1.4. Diagnosis:

1.4.1. During your stay:

The time between the appearance of the first symptom, the time between the first clinical sign and the diagnosis, and the time between the diagnosis and the resumption of surgery. The diagnosis is made on the ward or in intensive care. The length of stay in intensive care after bypass surgery.

1.4.1.1.   Causes of prolonged stays in intensive care :

Re-exploration, (circulatory assistance, re-intubation, ventilation time, pulmonary infection, respiratory distress, post-CEC cardiac dysfunction, (altered neurological status, development of sepsis, post-CEC atrial fibrillation and acute renal failure.

1.4.2. After discharge from hospital:

The time between discharge and onset of symptoms, the time between symptomatology and admission, the time between admission and recovery.

1.4.3. Diagnostic elements :

1.4.3.1.   Symptomatology :

Fever, chest pain, serositis or pus, scar inflammation, sternal instability, loss of skin substance. Occurrence of MI < 90 days, heart failure.

A critical state defined by cardiogenic shock, septic shock, severe sepsis, the use of catecholamines and circulatory assistance.

1.4.3.2.   Diagnosis:

Emergency degree: same-day resumption or deferred resumption.

Clinical diagnosis or imaging.

The identification of a germ in preoperative blood cultures or in a local sample in the event of a possibility of an infection.

1.4.3.3.   Premedication :

Preoperative antibiotic therapy and its duration, all causes combined.

1.4.3.4.   Biology :

Haemoglobin, white blood cell, CRP and procalcitonin levels.

2.   Per Operative Data :

2.1. Sternal closure techniques :

The number of steel wires, the closing technique: X, Simple, Frame.

The drainage system via thoracic drains or a thoracic Redon.

3.   Postoperative data :

3.1. Transfusion :

Total number of red blood cells per and post-op, post-op haemoglobin.

3.2. Post-recovery complications :

Re-examination, the need for circulatory assistance, the need for reintubation in the event of respiratory distress, the length of reintubation, pulmonary infection, cardiac dysfunction, altered neurological status, sepsis, acute renal failure.

3.3. Biology:

CRP and haemoglobin levels.

3.4. Bacteriological data :

The nature of the germ identified and the duration of antibiotic treatment.

3.5. Complications:

-    local complications: fistulation of the skin, discharge of pus or serositis, loss of skin substance.

-    Recurrence of mediastinitis.

-    Surgical revision.

3.6. Stay:

Length of stay in intensive care, length of postoperative stay, length of total hospitalisation.

4.   Mortality rate and cause of death :

8 Resume

Aim: To identify risk factors for mortality in patients with post cardiac surgery mediastinitis via sternotomy.

Methods: Retrospective study conducted in the cardiothoracic surgery department of the HMPIT between 1 January 2010 and 31 December 2019. The mediastinitis was defined as a deep infection of the operative site, requiring a surgical revision with positive bacteriological samples, or a macroscopic aspect of infection.

Risk factors for mortality were investigated on the basis of data relating to the patient, the initial surgery, the post-CEC operative follow-up, and the pre-, per- and post-operative management of the repeat surgery.

Results: 55 patients were included. The mortality rate in these patients was 30.9%.

the risk factors incriminated in the multivariate analysis were age over 60 and admission in a critical condition, as opposed to a preserved LVEF, which was a protective factor.

The most frequently identified microorganisms in bacteriological cultures were staphylococci, mainly aureus.

Conclusion:

A better understanding of the risk factors would enable appropriate measures to be taken to reduce the incidence of this infection, limit morbidity and mortality, and initiate preventive measures.

Key words	Mediastinitis, Mortality, Risk factors, Cardiac surgery, Adult, Sternotomy